AF683546

Beyond Boundaries of Biomedicine

Pragmatic Perspectives on Health and Disease

At the Interface

Dr Robert Fisher
Series Editor

Advisory Board

Professor Ned Basic
Professor James Cameron
Professor Margaret Chatterjee
Dr Salwa Ghaly
Professor Michael Goodman
Dr Diana Medlicott
Revd Stephen Morris
Professor John Parry
Dr David Seth Preston
Professor Dan Primozic
Revd Dr Kenneth Wilson, O.B.E

Volume 4

A volume in the *Probing the Boundaries* project
'Making Sense of: Health, Illness and Disease'

Probing the Boundaries

Beyond Boundaries of Biomedicine
Pragmatic Perspectives on Health and Disease

Wim J. van der Steen
Vincent K.Y. Ho
Ferry J. Karmelk

Rodopi

Amsterdam - New York, NY 2003

The paper on which this book is printed meets the requirements of "ISO 9706:1994, Information and documentation - Paper for documents - Requirements for permanence".

ISBN: 90-420-0816-4
©Editions Rodopi B.V., Amsterdam - New York, NY 2003
Printed in The Netherlands

About the Authors

Wim J. van der Steen, biologist and philosopher, is professor emeritus of philosophy of biology. He has worked at the Vrije Universiteit, Amsterdam, The Netherlands. He has published many books and articles in biology and philosophy of biology, medicine and philosophy of medicine, philosophy of science, and ethics.

Vincent K.Y. Ho, medical biologist, is a member of the program bureau of the Dutch Association of Comprehensive Cancer Centres (ACCC), Utrecht, The Netherlands, for the development and implementation of national oncological guidelines for treatment, nursing care and patient education. He is also a researcher in biomedicine. His publications include a book together with Wim J. van der Steen.

Ferry J. Karmelk, medical doctor and biologist, works at the psychiatric consortium Mediant, Enschede, The Netherlands.

We dedicate this book to three M's who mean much to us:

Mineke *Merel* *Marianne*

WJS
VKYH
FJK

Contents

Preface

Our book tells a story that is best assimilated by taking it in from the beginning to the end. As some of you may wish to read particular chapters only, we have tried to make the chapters self-contained and paid the price of being somewhat repetitious. Several themes, for example the role of omega-3 fatty acids in health and disease, and limitations of randomised controlled trials, recur in many chapters. But the context in which they are put is different in different chapters.

The book is out of the ordinary in that its prime target is missing knowledge rather than available knowledge. We are flooded nowadays with huge amounts of information from science, the media, and other sources. Literature in biomedicine is growing exponentially. Few researchers are in a position to oversee all sources of information that should be relevant to their specialism, since generalist work is being discouraged, in practice if not in principle. This conduces to the odd phenomenon of unconnected literatures that deal with similar subjects. We get to know more and more in some respects, but in other respects we get to know less and less. The existing body of knowledge is like a growing Swiss cheese. As you get more cheese, you also get more holes.

We aim to fill holes in current views of health and disease by a generalist approach that compensates for overspecialisation in biomedicine. But we would not endorse the ideal of an entirely solid cheese of future biomedical knowledge. Holes are unavoidable. The point is to get cheese and holes in the right places, in harmony with prevailing problems to be solved. We do hope that our own choice of cheese contributes to harmony for some readers.

Gratefully we thank colleagues who have helped us in our undertaking: Agostino di Giacomo Russo, David Healy, Artemis Simopoulos and Don Swanson. A grant from the Association for Christian Higher Education/Dittmer Foundation enabled VKYH to contribute to the book.

WJS
VKYH
FJK

Chapter 1

Introduction

The man was coughing again. Shocked he was as he discovered that his saliva had a reddish taint. Would he have a lung disease after all? Cancer perhaps? Long ago, relatives of his had died from LC, lung cancer. So he might be in danger. Scientists had discovered genes that increase the risk of contracting the disease, particularly for smokers. He did not smoke, but you never know. When he was young, he had lived in a town that was plagued by much air pollution, another risk factor. The coughing had begun after he lost his job and became depressed. His therapist had pointed out that this might impair his immune system—another risk factor. But the depression had only lasted for a few weeks. New antidepressives had put his brain to rest.

The saliva being what it was, he decided to consult his doctor at the BRS, the Body Repair Shop. After some tests, the doctor confirmed what he was afraid of: LC indeed. But no matter, even LC could mostly be cured now. Genes would have to be inserted in the program that had generated him, genes with chemical products that would destroy the cancer while leaving healthy tissues intact.

The war on cancer, heart disease and other non-infectious diseases had been won. Risks were now known beforehand by the genetic screening of embryos. If faulty genes were found, the embryo could be discarded, or improved by genetic modification. Infectious diseases had already disappeared in an earlier era. That had only been a matter of finding new drugs against microbes harming man. Also, the most dangerous microbes had been removed from the environment by sophisticated techniques. As environmental pollution was a thing of the past and

> *hamburgers had been replaced by new health foods, allergies had also disappeared.*
>
> *Some would complain that mental illnesses refused to go away. But that was only because many people refused to take medications that would change their brains toward pleasant moods and fitting behaviours.*
>
> *It is true that disease would often manage to slip through the net of constant vigilance cast widely by the medical profession. But seldom did that pose a problem, as medications could be targeted to remedy almost any malfunction.*

A weird story? Yes, would be our response. We would not bother you with it if everybody recognised it as science fiction. But, with a little bit less caricature, it is told in earnest even by many learned persons. Would it be possible for us to eradicate all diseases in the future, as new techniques will allow us to manipulate the human body away from misfortunes? There are those who manage to be that optimist. Schwartz (1998), a professor of medicine, is one of them:

> Exactly where we will stand in the war against disease by the year 2050 is of course impossible to say. But if developments in research maintain their current pace, it seems likely that a combination of improved attention to dietary and environmental factors along with advances in gene therapy and protein-targeted drugs will have virtually eliminated most major classes of disease. (Schwartz, 1998: 149)

But Schwartz does see a problem: the increase in numbers of human beings.

> ... thoughtful people have begun to consider medical advancement as a two-edged sword, not only because of the economic consequences ... but also because it threatens to distort the natural cycle of birth, aging and death. Although restrictions on reproductive freedom or a mandated approach to euthanasia may today seem unthinkable, in another fifty years the severity of the population problem may be such that all conceivable solutions will be on the table. (Schwartz,

> 1998: 155)

We do hope that persons such as Schwartz will not become a major force in politics. His optimism is anyhow without warrant. Considering drugs, we regard his optimism as an example of the magic bullet fallacy:

> The magic bullet fallacy
>
> When new drugs are first introduced their introduction is usually accompanied by glowing accounts which stress their effectiveness and their freedom from side effects. Such optimism is falsely grounded because any drug which interferes with the biochemistry of the human organism must have undesirable effects. Experience quickly teaches that the drugs are not as effective as first thought and that their use is by no means trouble free. (Skrabanek and McCormick, 1989: 38)

Schwartz also underestimates the extent of human shortcomings. Medical professionals have shortcomings like everybody else. Some have indeed argued that, with respect to errors, the medical profession compares unfavourably with other professions. Medicine has not developed effective strategies of error prevention. Leape (1999), who illustrates the absence of effective strategies with examples from a large literature, argues that the reasons for this situation are to be found in the culture of medical practice. Physicians are socialised to strive for error-free practice, and they tend to emphasise perfection in diagnosis and treatment (an emphasis that accords well with the vision of Schwartz). This works against openness about mistakes. Also, physicians have to face the malpractice threat that may put their career in jeopardy.

> One study of errors in a medical intensive care unit revealed an average of 1.7 errors per day per patient ... . (...) Given the complex nature of medical practice and the multitude of interventions that each patient receives, a high error rate is perhaps not surprising. The patients in the intensive care unit study, for example, were the recipients of an average of 178 'activities' per day. The 1.7 errors per day thus indicate that hospital personnel were functioning at a 99 per cent level of proficiency. However, a 1 per cent failure rate is

> substantially higher than is tolerated in industry, particularly in hazardous fields such as aviation and nuclear power. As Deming (1987) points out, even 99.9 per cent may not be good enough: 'If we had to live with 99.9 per cent, we would have [in the United States]: two unsafe plane landings per day at O'Hare, 16,000 pieces of lost mail every hour, 32,000 bank checks deducted from the wrong bank account every hour.' (Leape 1999: 21)

With Leape, we assume that a decrease of medical errors should be possible. But it would be unrealistic to assume that patient landings could become as safe as plane landings. Patients are organisms, and organisms are much more complex than planes. Handling them is therefore a risky affair. Furthermore, you cannot pull organisms apart and then put them together again. With machines, such a thing is often possible. Organisms die if you start pulling them apart.

In his book, Schwartz disregards ecology, the science that studies relationships between organisms and environments. We conjecture that this oversight is at the root of his excessive optimism. We illustrate the dangers of this kind of optimism by a brief case study of malaria. This infectious disease is caused by a parasite which is transmitted to human beings by several species of mosquitoes. Malaria-control strategies aim at the eradication of the mosquitoes and at prevention and cure by medication.

Garrett (1994), in a deservedly well-known book, has warned us against the naive assumption that medicine has in principle won the battle against infectious diseases (see also the more recent book by Price-Smith, 2002, who has a similar message). The diseases are making a comeback. That was to be expected. Insights from ecology and other subdisciplines of biology pointed in this direction, but medical professionals did not take heed as they had no adequate knowledge of ecology.

> For Western physicians, the 1950s and 1960s were a time of tremendous optimism. Nearly every week the medical establishment declared another "miracle breakthrough" in humanity's war with infectious disease. Antibiotics, first discovered in the 1940s, were now growing in number and potency. (...) Medicine was viewed as a huge chart depicting disease incidences over time: by the twenty-first century every infectious disease on the chart would have hit zero. Few scientists or

> physicians of the day doubted that humanity would continue on its linear course of triumphs over the microbes. (Garrett, 1994: 30)

The World Health Organisation assumed that malaria would soon cease to be of major importance. Pesticides would wipe out the mosquitoes transmitting it. In 1955, the Eighth World Health Assembly voted to initiate a program for the global eradication of malaria. This represented a remarkable leap of faith. Many health authorities, both within and outside the Assembly, viewed eradication as at best fool-hardy, and at worst, potentially disastrous (Packard, 1998). Their warnings were disregarded.

This was the Age of Boosterism. The notion developed of a Health Transition, as it was called (Garrett, 1994: 31).

> What would remain were the slower chronic diseases that primarily struck in old age, particularly cancer and heart disease. Everybody would live longer, disease-free lives. (Garrett, 1994: 32)
>
> Boosters of the 1950s and early 1960s had some basis, born of ignorance, for their optimism: they knew comparatively little about genetics, microbial evolution, the human immune system, or disease ecology. Given the state of knowledge in the public health world of that day, it may have seemed appropriate to view infectious diseases in simple cause-and-effect terms. Seen in such a reductionist manner, problems and solutions appeared obvious and readily conquerable, bravado warranted. (idem: 33)

Humanity's great success story would be smallpox. But a very different outcome awaited those who fought to eradicate malaria. After initial successes, malaria started to increase again during the 1960s. The Green Revolution, financed by the World Bank, was getting underway. Monocultured farms took the place of areas with diverse plant life. Pesticides were needed to protect the crops against insects, which now had fewer natural enemies. Then insect resistance against antibiotics became a major problem so that croplands could be overwhelmed rapidly by destructive insects.

> Farmers responded during the 1960s with heavy pesticide use, which often worked in the short

> term. But in the long run pesticides usually killed off beneficial insects, while the crop-attacking pests became resistant to chemicals.
>
> At the very time malaria control efforts were splintering or collapsing, the agricultural use of DDT and its sister compounds was soaring. Almost overnight resistant mosquito populations appeared all over the world. (Garrett, 1994: 51)

Resistance against drugs also developed.

> Increasingly the experts saw the grand smallpox success as an aberration, rather than a goal that could easily be replicated with other diseases.
>
> In 1975 the worldwide incidence of malaria was about 2.5 times what it had been in 1961 .... (...) A new global iatrogenic form of malaria was emerging—“iatrogenic” meaning created as a result of medical treatment. In its well-meaning zeal to treat the world’s malaria scourge, humanity had created a new epidemic. (Garrett, 1994: 52)

If anything, the situation became even worse after the appearance of Garrett’s book in 1994. Some 500,000,000 persons are suffering from malaria. Resistance of the parasite against insecticides has contributed to a marked increase of malaria, in Africa for example (Trape *et al.*, 2002). New medications have been developed, but resistance may develop against them as well. Combination therapies involving unrelated drugs may be successful (Nosten and Brasseur, 2002). But the parasite is versatile: multidrug resistance is a problem in several regions (Wongsrichanalai *et al.*, 2002).

The problem is made worse by an inadequate eradication strategy. The current strategy emphasises insecticides against adult mosquitoes. It is not very successful as the mosquitoes easily develop resistance. Killeen *et al.* (2002) point out that campaigns against the mosquitoes have been the most successful in the 1930s and 1940s, locally in Brazil, Egypt and Zambia. The success was achieved through an integrated programme that relied overwhelmingly upon larval control. After the advent of the insecticide DDT this approach was neglected and global malaria-control policy shifted toward the control of adult mosquitoes. Larval-control methods should now be reprioritised as an additional way to roll back malaria.

Joint efforts of organisations and industries involved are needed to get effective antimalarial strategies off the ground. Unfortunately, such efforts are rare. Hardwicke (2002) notes that no article published in the scientific press in the last 10 years reviews areas of interest common to the World Health Organisation (WHO) and the pharmaceutical industry. The WHO itself does not function optimally. Horton (2002) states that its leadership is unwilling to address tensions within the organisation caused by poor management.

Malaria is obviously not a subject to be grasped by medical research on its own. Nor would it be reasonable to relegate the entire search for treatments to medicine. Many disciplines have a significant bearing on malaria. For example, insights from evolutionary biology are valuable as mosquito evolution determines epidemiological patterns (Carter and Mendis, 2002; Killeen *et al.*, 2002; Hartl *et al.*, 2002). We also need contributions from political and social science, economy, and agricultural science. For example, Singer and De Castro (2001) have shown that malaria transmission on the Amazon frontier depends on macropolitical, social and economic policies, human migration and agricultural development. Garfield (1999) has a similar message concerning Nicaragua. In that country, an antimalarial strategy based on frequent local epidemiological assessments and community participation was developed in the 1980s. But the expected improvements did not occur. Nicaragua experienced its worst epidemics in the 1990s, caused in part by malfunctioning health care. The country's macroeconomic structural adjustment programme, established after the contra war, decreased the motivation of volunteers and malaria control workers.

In brief, research on malaria and antimalarial strategies need resources from many disciplines of science. Our first priority should be to get the resources in a balanced perspective. We can but improve on the existing situation if we stop feeding optimism with one-sided science.

Modern science should not be our sole source of information. Indigenous folk medicine is also an important source of knowledge in the search for new drugs. Recent research has demonstrated antimalarial activity of medicinal plants from many tropical countries (Tona *et al.*, 1999: Congo; Willcox, 1999: Uganda; Marshall *et al.*, 2000: Sierra Leone; Munoz *et al.*, 2000a: Bolivia, Altenos Indians; Munoz *et al.*, 2000b: Bolivia, Chacobo Indians; Mustofa *et al.*, 2000: Ivory Coast; Oketch-Rabah *et al.*, 2000: Kenya; Addae-Kyereme *et al.*, 2001: Ghana; Deharo *et al.*, 2001: Bolivia, Tacana Indians). The value of traditional knowledge of malaria is now being recognised. In 1999, the first international meeting of the Research Initiative on Traditional Antimalarial Methods (RITAM) was held in Nairobi, hosted by the Global Initiative for Traditional Systems of

Health (GIFTS) at Oxford University and the WHO (Bodeker and Willcox, 2000).

The case of malaria exhibits major themes that play a role throughout our book (numbers after examples refer to chapters and sections):

- *Medicine must move beyond its current boundaries.* The case of malaria shows that medicine has still to assimilate insights from several subdisciplines of biology such as ecology. The existing boundaries are restrictive, since medicine focuses on a limited area of biology. To understand diseases, we also have to reckon with disciplines at a farther remove from medicine: sociology, political science, anthropology, and so forth. It would be unreasonable to demand that medical professionals acquire full expertise in these disciplines. But if they ignore them, they may end up with inadequate theories and inadequate medical treatments. We would plead for a change of culture that de-emphasises roles of disciplines. The emphasis should rather be on problems, for example the problem of how to deal with malaria. Some health problems call for the use of materials from many disciplines, to be integrated in interdisciplinary, generalist studies. Theorising within the boundaries of biomedicine has its uses, but relative to many health problems it is obsolete.
  Text with examples. All the chapters contain examples, but some chapters (3, 10 and 11) have varieties of this theme as the main subject.

- *Missing stuffs and arrows (MSA) are unavoidable in medicine.* This is a corollary of the previous theme. *MSA* is an expression of our own that needs some clarification. It applies in a literal way, for example, to diagrams of metabolic pathways with arrows representing causal links of conversion among substances. Diagrams are necessarily incomplete. Stuffs and arrows have to be missing as we cannot represent them all. If we are not aware of this, we run the risk of staying with one-sided theories. Metaphorically, we also use the expression *MSA* for missing theories or even entire disciplines, and relations among them. In the study of malaria, ecology and relations between ecological factors and the disease represented *MSA*. We see many *MSA* as missed opportunities.
  Text with examples. Our entire approach amounts to a search for

opportunities missed by mainstream research and mainstream therapies. Varieties of *MSA* play a role in all the chapters, implicitly or explicitly.

- *Overmedication is common.* Medications that have been used against malaria were effective in themselves. However, their use on a massive scale has invited disaster. The disasters were not foreseen by medical professionals as they lacked ecological insights. Examples also exist of massive medication that is hardly effective and dangerous at that. Case studies in several chapters indicate that this situation is maintained to a great extent by the pharmaceutical industry. Hence the next theme.
  Text with examples. Psychotropic drugs (4.3, 6.3, 6.4, 10.2 and 10.3), antacids such as omeprazole and antibiotics (8.1 and 8.3), NSAIDs, non-steroid anti-inflammatory drugs (8.2).

- *Commercial interests in medicine should be kept in check.* The industry makes huge profits from overmedication. In the case of malaria, drugs may have been effective in themselves. But the way they were used resulted in disasters. It is desirable that we effect a regulation of drugs by persons and organisations without direct or indirect interests in marketing. Politicians often collaborate with the industry. This enhances inadequate drug regulation. Politics has to be controlled by independent authorities to avoid bias.
  Text with examples. See the previous theme; several chapters provide detailed comments concerning the industry (6.3 and 8.2) and politics (3.3, 3.4, 6.3, 7.3 and 8.2).

- *Existing boundaries between regular and alternative medicine must be reassessed.* In the case of malaria, evidence shows that many valuable indigenous medications exist. Once proven effective, they may be passed on to regular medicine. We plead for openness in medicine toward sources of knowledge outside the domain of "normal" science. Foreign ideas have to be tested in some way, but they should not be rejected in a dogmatic *a priori* fashion.
  Text with examples. Cancer (4.5), general considerations (11).

Two additional themes, which are less salient in the malaria case, play major roles in the book:

- *Randomised controlled trials (RCTs) are overvalued.* A recent, now dominant paradigm of medicine goes by the name of "Evidence-Based Medicine." The name is odd, because it appears to express the obvious. However, "evidence" is used here in a narrow sense, with much emphasis on a quantitative method for testing medical treatments: RCTs. We oppose undue emphasis on RCTs and quantitative methods in general, which have many limitations, and we plead for generalist approaches that draw on a great variety of evidence.
  Text with examples. RCTs are a theme in many chapters (3.2, 4.2, 4.3, 5.4, 6.3, 8.2, 9, 10.2 and 10.6).

- *Diet therapies are undervalued in medicine.* We argue in several chapters that many diets in civilised countries are deficient in omega-3 fatty acids. This fosters chronic diseases and psychiatric disorders. Omega-3 fatty acids used as food supplements help prevent many diseases, and they also have curative effects. Diet therapies could presumably outperform drug therapies in many cases.
  Text with examples. Treatments with omega-3 polyunsaturated fatty acids (PUFAs) are considered in several chapters (3.2, 5.6, 7.3, 7.4, 8.4, 10.4, 10.5 and 10.6).

We apply the seven themes to somatic diseases and also to mental disorders. The boundary between the two categories is problematic. Also problematic is the boundary between mental disorders and human suffering. We address these boundary problems in several chapters.

Chapters 2-4 set the stage by general comments on the diagnosis and the classification of diseases (2), causes of disease, particularly environmental causes (3), and the role of RCTs in the assessment of medical treatments (4). Chapter 5 is a detailed case study of migraine. In Chapter 6 we analyse limitations of psychiatry, especially biological psychiatry. Chapters 7-10 deal with the role of omega-3 fatty acids in health and disease (general overview: 7; rheumatoid arthritis and stomach ulcers: 8 and 9; mental illnesses: 10). Chapters 11 and 12 put medicine in a broader context by a comparison of conventional approaches with CAM, complementary and alternative medicine (Chapter 11), and case studies concerning medicine and religion (Chapter 12).

Appendix 1 provides chapter summaries in greater detail. In Appendix 2 we review genetics and philosophy of biology. These disciplines get little explicit attention in the book, but they are important as a background. Philosophy of medicine is less relevant for us, since it is not as much concerned with live science in progress at the level of primary sources.

Genetics is now at the forefront of biomedicine, and knowledge of genetic factors underlying diseases allows of beneficial applications in some cases. But the existing emphasis on genetics detracts from environmental causes of disease. We do not extensively partake of ongoing disputes about the merits of genetic approaches, but focus on influences of environmental factors on health and disease that are often disregarded.

Philosophy of biology is not an explicit subject in the book for a different reason. During the last few decades, many excellent texts have been published by philosophers of biology. In principle, they can help us assess research in biology and biomedicine. However, the texts are generally at an advanced level, and they often concentrate on a limited area of biology, evolutionary biology and, to a lesser extent, neuroscience. We feel that philosophy at the more elementary level of plain logic should be our first concern in the appraisal of ongoing biomedical research. Philosophers of biology mostly leave the logic of science to researchers in biology and biomedicine, but these researchers, unlike psychologists for example, seldom bother about the logic of science.

One of us has published a practical primer that bridges the gap between advanced level philosophy and research in biology and biomedicine, with a great variety of examples from live science and exercises (Van der Steen, 1993a). In Van der Steen and Ho (2001a) the practical approach is applied to analysis of literature in the life sciences (for a similar approach of the life sciences in the context of ethics, see Van der Steen, 1995, 1999b; Van der Steen and Ho, 2001a). We follow the lead of this book by logical analyses of texts. Such analyses often bring to the surface an amazing variety of covert assumptions that are easily overlooked.

Appendix 1 to Chapter 1

Summary of the Book

Chapter 2 introduces medicine's approach of diseases. Medicine does not have a single unifying theory of disease. Nor does it have a single overarching concept of disease. That is because the category of diseases is heterogeneous. Heterogeneity also exists within diseases we care to distinguish, owing to biological variability. Thus, all classifications of diseases have to be arbitrary to some extent (Section 2). We illustrate the heterogeneity among and within diseases by representative examples: muscle diseases, fibromyalgia, the chronic fatigue syndrome and rheumatoid arthritis (Section 3).

Classifications of aetiological factors (causes of disease) are often incomplete. For example, the common amalgamation of two dichotomies, internal *versus* external causes and biological *versus* psychosocial causes, leaves out external biological factors as studied by ecology (Section 2). This kind of classification is associated with much emphasis in medicine on genetics and molecular biology, at the cost of ecological factors such as diet (Section 3).

Psychological factors play important roles in many diseases, but the "biomedical model" in medicine, with its emphasis on the body, cannot accommodate psychological factors in a satisfactory way (Section 2). This may invite a fallacious labelling of diseases without known somatic causes (fibromyalgia for example) as "psychogenic" (Section 3).

Chapter 3 deals with causes of diseases and treatments, the emphasis being on environmental factors, in particular biological, social and political factors that are often disregarded in mainstream medicine.

Deficiencies of omega-3 PUFAs (polyunsaturated fatty acids) contribute to many diseases in our culture (Section 2). Dietary treatments with these acids could outperform drug therapies in many cases. Evolutionary theory helps us understand the causes of the deficiencies and the rationale of the treatments. These things are not recognised in many areas of medicine. We describe a single-case study of a schizophrenia patient who recovered after omega-3 treatment. The study has implications for Evidence-Based Medicine with its gold standard of randomised controlled trials (RCTs, the subject of Chapter 4). Several features of the study (spectacular cure, failure of other treatments, a theory explaining the outcome) impart on it an evidential force that compares favourably with many RCTs.

A case study of tuberculosis shows that models of epidemiology and of social science do not explain drug resistance in this illness in a satisfactory way (Section 3). Existing scientific explanations are inadequate as they overlook the role of structural violence against the poor in some regions.

A case study of air pollution also concerns poverty as a significant cause of disease (Section 4). Contrary to common wisdom, the study demonstrates that pollution risks may reinforce rather than cut across class inequalities. Politicians, in the case at hand, denied this by a distortion of evidence.

Chapter 4 reviews strong and weak points of RCTs, the primary stronghold of Evidence-Based Medicine. In RCTs, effects of medical treatments are assessed by a comparison with placebo treatments. Thus, drugs are to be compared with substances that do not have the effects attributed to the drugs. Ideal RCTs have a double-blind set-up, both the doctors and the patients being "blind" in that they do not know who is receiving the genuine treatment. Even this ideal set-up has many potential shortcomings, some of them unavoidable (Section 2). For example, the samples of patients studied have to meet strict criteria that make them unrepresentative of the population to be studied. We face here the paradox that scientific adequacy may be at odds with clinical relevance.

Another fundamental problem has to do with unavoidable selectivity (Section 1). For example, the observation that patients receiving a drug are better off overall than patients receiving a placebo need not imply that the drug represents the best treatment. Treatments which are disregarded in an RCT could outperform the treatments studied. A case study concerning treatments of mental illness with psychotropic drugs or psychotherapy illustrates the problem (Section 3). The drugs are often prescribed on the basis of problematic RCTs. Evidence suggests that psychotherapy is to be preferred to drug therapy in many cases. But psychotherapies also have problematic features (Section 4). Beneficial effects of such therapies appear to be caused by non-specific factors, for example humane contact, which can also be provided by laypersons. Indeed, the formal expertise of therapists is unrelated to therapeutic success.

The last section of the chapter (Section 5) is a case study of cancer focussing on psychosocial treatment modes and complementary and alternative medicine (CAM). The influence of psychosocial factors in cancer is controversial. Research on the value of CAM treatments has faced political obstruction. A valuable old cancer therapy based on the principle that bacterial infection may effect cures, has almost faded into oblivion.

Chapter 5 is an extensive case study of migraine that illustrates all the points made in previous chapters. To start with, we focus on the massive growth of literature in biomedicine, which results in specialisms without optimal connections (Section 1). Migraine is a disorder which cannot be understood without an integration of resources from many disciplines. It is in fact a heterogeneous collection of conditions that preclude neat classification (Section 2). Theories of migraine concentrate with different emphases on blood circulation, the nervous system, hormones and the immune system (Section 3). Many drug treatments for migraine are available, but no drug works for all patients. Owing to the heterogeneity of migraine phenomena, treatments have to be individualised, and the clinical relevance of drug assessment with RCTs is limited for this reason (Section 4).

We present ideas about migraine that are missing in mainstream medicine, which may help us find new treatments. Common sense, elementary biology and anecdotal observations by one of us indicate that the general blood circulation may be influenced by exercise and massage so as to prevent or abate migraine attacks (Section 5). Also, we have formulated a new hypothesis based on indirect evidence in the literature, which suggests that the hormone vasopressin should play a crucial role in migraine (Section 6). It is amazing that almost all research on hormones and hormone-like substances affecting migraine has been done about serotonin. As hormones interact, the idea that one hormone should be that important is implausible. Indirect evidence obtained from the literature also suggests that deficiencies of omega-3 PUFAs may play a role in migraine.

Next, we argue that research on migraine neglects higher levels of organisation. Also, evolutionary biology and functional biology merit more attention (Sections 7 and 8). All in all, the existing literature on migraine, however extensive, disregards many possibilities to improve on existing theories and treatments.

Chapter 6 is a critical survey of psychiatry, especially biological psychiatry. The discipline is problematic for a variety of reasons (Section 1). It lacks a solid foundation because we do not have a satisfactory theory to explain relations between the mental and the physical. Existing classifications of mental illnesses are controversial, and the boundary between mental illness and ordinary suffering is diffuse. The tendency exists to attribute mental problems to biological pathology when biological correlates are found, but this represents a fallacy.

We review valuable recent analyses of the situation in biological psychiatry by Boyle (2002) (Section 2) and Healy (2002) (Section 3). An analysis of other sources confirms their views, which are extremely critical (Section 4). The Diagnostic and Statistical Manual of Mental Disorders (DSM), the classification of mental disorders used by many psychiatrists, is way below standards of good science. For example, Boyle shows convincingly that schizophrenia defined as in successive versions of the DSM has no foothold in reality. Healy observes that the pharmaceutical industry has influenced theorising in psychiatry in a negative way, and that it has managed to market ineffective drugs with dangerous side effects on a massive scale. He also argues that Evidence-Based Medicine is overvalued in psychiatry at the cost of clinical judgments.

We conjecture that elementary biology disregarded in current research on mental illnesses may help us find new treatments, as in the case of migraine. A brief case study of anorexia nervosa illustrates this. Positive outcomes have been obtained with a therapy centring on temperature regulation (Section 5). Therapies in mainstream psychiatry have overlooked the crucial role of body temperature in anorexia.

In conclusion, we argue that psychiatry is in a difficult position because it is made responsible for social ills of society (Section 6).

Chapter 7 reviews deficiencies of omega-3 PUFAs in modern diets, which contribute to many diseases. Official nutrition guidelines do not adequately account for these deficiencies, and the pharmaceutical industry, which understandably funds research on drug therapies rather than diet therapies, also contributes to this situation (Section 1). Official approaches of diet have long harped on the lowering of (some varieties of) blood cholesterol, but the cholesterol story is a myth rather than good science (Section 2).

Literature in many disciplines outside mainstream medicine confirms the importance of omega-3 deficiencies (Section 3). Food companies are also focussing on the deficiencies, and they market new products containing omega-3 PUFAs, but the arguments they present are less solid. This creates problems, as authorities regulating the food companies have opposed the arguments while disregarding good evidence.

Several studies that put the omega-3 issue in the context of evolutionary biology and several other disciplines have shown that the deficiencies are implicated in cancers and heart disease (Section 4).

Chapter 8 analyses the role of omega-3 deficiencies in autoimmune diseases and gastric ulcers. We argue that these conditions are overmedicated, and that the alternative of diet therapies calls for more research.

An example concerning an expensive drug, omeprazole (Losec), illustrates overmedication reinforced by politics (Section 1). The drug is an antacid which reduces the acidity of the stomach. It is used in huge quantities to treat gastrointestinal disorders—ulcers and milder conditions.

Next, we review the use of non-steroid anti-inflammatory drugs (NSAIDs), which are primarily used to treat autoimmune disorders such as rheumatoid arthritis (Section 2). These drugs are also used increasingly against all sorts of aches. NSAIDs often have serious side effects, for example gastric ulcers, which invites the use of omeprazole on top of the NSAIDs. NSAIDs are even responsible for a considerable mortality. The marketing of NSAIDs has often been based on biased RCTs without much evidential forces funded by the pharmaceutical industry. Moreover, authorities responsible for regulation have sided with the industry in irresponsible ways.

Gastric ulcers may be caused by NSAIDs, but also by infection with the bacterium *Helicobacter pylori* (Section 3). *H. pylori* infections are often treated with omeprazole or another antacid together with antibiotics. But the treatment does not always work, it has side effects, and antibiotic resistance of bacteria is becoming an ever more serious problem.

It is unfortunate that the alternative of diet treatments with omega-3 PUFAs has been pushed to the margins of research. These treatments may be far the best way to prevent autoimmune diseases and gastrointestinal disorders (Section 4).

The philosopher Thagard (1999) has published an extensive historical analysis of research that puts *H. pylori* on the scene as a salient cause of gastric ulcers. He reconstructs biomedical theorising about the issue as an eminently rational affair (Section 5). As Thagard understandably sides with mainstream research in medicine, he reinforces the existing bias which privileges drug therapies over diet therapies. Methods of Evidence-Based Medicine enhance this bias as they are implemented in disregard of dietary deficiencies.

Chapter 9 is a continuation of the case studies in Chapter 8, with a somewhat different emphasis. We argue that Evidence-Based Medicine, however useful, obscures from us the need of qualitative in addition to quantitative research methods. To make this point, we compare risk assessments with RCTs (Sections 2 and 3). Both methods are geared to the analysis of alternative options that do not exhaust the possibilities. That is why they have to be supplemented with qualitative approaches. The point is reinforced by views of researchers in "qualitative science" (Section 4).

Additional comments on RCTs strengthen points made in previous chapters (Sections 4 and 5). The crucial idea is that our methods of investigation cannot comply with all methodological criteria which are reasonable in themselves. For example, RCTs which are set up in a rigorous way necessarily use patient samples that are not representative for the population we wish to study. Thus, rigor does not sit well with clinical relevance. This is a so-called trade-off problem. In doing statistical analyses, we also face trade-offs, because we cannot at the same time minimise the error of rejecting a true hypothesis and the error of accepting a false hypothesis. So we have to decide which kind of error is the most important for us. As the interests of drug companies and the interests of patients are associated with different errors, our decision determines what interests we serve.

These dilemmas obviously cannot be solved by quantitative methods. Indeed, they cannot be solved by scientific means. In conclusion, Evidence-Based Medicine cannot stand on its own. It has to be supplemented with qualitative considerations that ultimately rely on ethics, and on common sense.

Chapter 10, like Chapter 8, is an inquiry into diet treatments with omega-3 PUFAs as an alternative to drug treatments. Mental illnesses are now our subject. We argue that recorded prevalences of these illnesses are implausibly high, that problems of daily life are often construed as mental illnesses, that overmedication with psychotropic drugs is common, and that the pharmaceutical industry is responsible for biased RCTs that enhance overmedication (Section 2).

We subsequently analyse a common type of fallacious argument designed to attribute mental illness to biological pathology (Section 3). If a drug alleviates mental symptoms and also has an effect on the brain in persons with the symptoms, we are not allowed to infer that something is wrong with the brain of these persons. This line of reasoning is one among many examples of bad science pushing psychiatry toward a restrictive biological approach.

Recent research indicates that omega-3 PUFAs are a promising treatment option for psychiatry (Sections 4, 5 and 6). As yet, studies of drug treatments vastly outnumber studies of diet treatments. A change of emphasis is badly needed, but this is difficult to achieve since funding by the industry privileges drug therapies.

In conclusion, we argue that psychiatry needs resources from many disciplines to overcome restrictive approaches of mental illnesses (Section 7).

Chapter 11 deals with the dichotomy of conventional medicine and CAM (complementary and alternative medicine). We regard the dichotomy as outdated. First, we show that boundaries between disciplines have become elusive. Like diseases, disciplines are to large extent arbitrary entities (Section 1). Next, we review materials from previous chapters which jointly show that the existing boundaries of medicine are restrictive. To the extent that we restrict medical science to biology, we get bad science (Section 2).

We argue that conventional approaches and approaches in CAM have different strengths and weaknesses (Sections 3 and 4). The assumption that conventional medicine is the better option because it is evidence-based, which CAM is not, is simplistic. The signs are that some CAM therapies are promising, but evidence in favour of these therapies is still limited. Conventional medicine should assimilate proven therapies from CAM. This is not to say that theories from CAM are to be assimilated at the same time. At the level of theories and worldviews, links between conventional medicine and CAM are not easily forged.

Chapter 12 puts medicine in the context of religion. To set the stage, we review literature dealing with relations between the mental and the physical (Section 1). Next, we analyse two extreme views on relations between biomedical science and religion (Section 2). Some defend the view that the study of brain processes in persons doing meditation may help us justify a religious worldview. We regard this as an ambitious undertaking. Another extreme view construes research that aims at theories overarching religion and medicine as a venture without merit. Thus, effects of prayer or distant healing on health could not be investigated in a scientifically responsible way. We regard this view as overly pessimistic. An autobiographical example of anecdotal evidence in favour of distant healing shows that research into the issue should be feasible.

We also analyse opposing views about NDEs, near-death experiences (Section 3). Some researchers interpret these experiences in materialistic terms. They regard them as symptoms of brain malfunction. Our analysis indicates that this view is simplistic and unconvincing. Others interpret NDEs as religious experiences of a spiritual world encountered by a "soul" or "spirit" that can leave the body. We see no reason for an *a priori* rejection of this possibility. Conceivably, further studies of NDEs may help to make it plausible.

Appendix 2 to Chapter 1

Genetics and Philosophy of Biology

Research on "disease genes" is mostly done in disregard of many social and other environmental factors known to affect health. The hypothetical scenario that follows reveals that this generates biased views.

We decide to study depression in persons who are afflicted by poverty. A thousand persons who are severely depressed are subjected to genetic screening. Another thousand persons in similar conditions of poverty but without depression serve as controls. We discover that the depressed persons have particular combinations of genes that are missing in the controls. Furthermore, we discover that the gene combinations are associated with particular features of the brain. If these features are induced in animals by artificial means, they provoke behaviours that resemble behaviours of depressed persons. What more could we want? We have demonstrated that depression is caused by genetic factors, and it stands to reason that the most promising treatments should be medications that bring the observed pathological features of the brain back to normal, or gene therapies that compensate for the aberrations.

In another study, we do the same screening with similar persons, but during a period of a few months beforehand, we provide the subjects with money to alleviate their poverty so that they can eat well. Now we get a different result. The genetic differences between the groups are the same as in the previous study, but the depressed persons get well before the screening is done, and we do not find differences between the two groups in brain features.

The lesson should be clear: The effects of genes depend on the context. If we study genes in a particular context, then our results are valid only for this context. In rare cases, effects may occur across many different contexts. That, and only that, would be a reason to allot special significance to genes (for details concerning this point of logic, see Van der Steen, 1999a). It is difficult to get this point in the right perspective, since research on "disease genes" is funded to excess, whereas research on contextual factors such as poverty and food has been pushed to the margin. Well, if we keep doing genetic research, then we will get genetic results. But if our research is limited to genetics, then we will not know what our results mean in a broader context.

The growth of genetic investigations into human diseases is well reflected by the growth of *The metabolic and molecular bases of inherited disease* (Scriver *et al.*, 2001); the 8th edition is a four-volume set with 5,570 pages. This is an immensely valuable store of knowledge. But where is it leading? Childs (1999), in commenting on the 7th edition, sees the new genetics of disease as a welcome development. He notes that all diseases are going to be seen as inherited, while granting that the environment is equally important. The new approach accounts for genetic variability. That is an asset. We wonder though, how the new system is to be combined, say, with nutritional approaches. The 9th edition of *Modern nutrition in health and disease* (Shils *et al.*, 1999), which merely has 1,951 pages, contains a rich store of data on nutrients affecting diseases. Many of the diseases are also in the text by Scriver *et al.* For the rest, the two texts have little in common. Other texts on nutrition, metabolism and disease (Groff *et al.*, 1995; Morrison and Hark, 1999; Bender, 2002) also have few links with genetics. We do not see how Scriver *et al.*, whose undertaking is already immense, could accommodate all available information about nutrition (and all sorts of environmental factors) in their classification of disorders. If we make genetics the measure of classification, environmental approaches are easily undervalued. The chances are that some persons suffering from a dietary deficiency will then be diagnosed as having an inherited disorder. We somehow have to find a generalist approach that does not make genetics the primary measure of all things (in biology, the approach of Burdon, 1999, who integrates genetics with environmental studies, is a good starting point).

Research into the genetics of psychological features and behaviours deserves special scrutiny, because it is plagued by enduring controversies, about the nature of mental illnesses for example (for criticism of undue emphasis on genes in these illnesses, see Kaplan, 2000). Disputes about the genetics of intelligence show most clearly that this research affects culture in profound ways. There are those who, assuming that intelligence has a considerable genetic component, justify existing social inequalities on the ground that they are natural. A book by Herrnstein and Murray (1994) is well-known for taking this stance. They argue that intelligence is genetically determined to a great extent, and that black persons are on average much less intelligent than white persons owing to their genetic make-up. Their message is an old one: Human misery is natural, inequality is fated and, owing to native talents, humans deserve the positions they have in society.

The authors' notion of genetic determination endorsed is flawed because they—and many others with them—are confusing it with heritability, which is an entirely different notion. Richardson (1999) explains the issue in an accessible way:

> Most people will have heard or read that [the] nature—nurture debate is about the heritability of IQ. They will probably interpret this to mean the extent to which IQ is inherited or genetically determined. This is a rather sloppy kind of understanding of heritability that is often, unfortunately, slipped into by those who should know better. Heritability, indeed, has a very restricted meaning: it is an estimate of the degree of overall variation in a character in a sample or population that is associated with genetic differences in the same population in the particular environments, in which the sample is living at that time.
>
> It is now widely acknowledged that a heritability estimate cannot apply to any other population (in a different set of circumstances or the same population at a different time), and that it can not predict the consequences of any kind of intervention. (Richardson, 1999: 74)

The confusion described by Richardson concerns context-dependence as revealed by our hypothetical study of depression. Richardson shows that leading researchers investigating the genetics of intelligence (and the genetics of mental faculties and behaviour in general) know about it. Yet they often succumb to fallacious inferences from heritability towards genetic determination. The same situation exists in research on mental illnesses (Kaplan, 2000).

Itzkoff (1994) has a message that resembles that of Herrnstein and Murray. He envisages more daring implications of research on intelligence, as he worries about a putative decline of overall intelligence in America. One of his recommendations to counteract the decline is to persuade potentially parasitic persons at the bottom of society to refrain from conceiving and having children—for one generation (Itzkoff, 1994: 195). His view, like that of Herrnstein and Murray, presupposes genetic determination, without any evidence (for additional critical comments concerning the genetics of intelligence, see Nelkin and Lindee, 1995; Fischer *et al.*,1996; Howe, 1997; Mackintosh, 1998).

The most deplorable aspect of this kind of work is its common emphasis on differences between races (a main theme of Herrnstein and

Murray, not as obviously Itzkoff), which easily invites racism. The most extensive survey of racial differences is by Rushton (1997). On the basis of data interpreted by the aid of evolutionary biology, he defends the view that genetic differences between races in intelligence, brain and behaviour are profound. But solid genetic evidence is almost lacking in his book. The entire enterprise is suspect because the idea that races should be different genetically is a non-starter. Some differences exist, but genetic differences among individuals within populations vastly exceed differences between populations (Cavalli-Sforza, 2000).

Marriages of evolutionary theory and genetics that trivialise the role of the environment have tended towards eugenics and racism for a long time. The present marriage does not have the blessing of biology beyond the narrow confines of "geneticism"; for critical comments we refer to a sample of good books: Shipman (1994), Caudill (1997), Sykes (1999), Dugatkin (2000) and Segerstråle (2000).

The young discipline of evolutionary psychology is entirely devoted to the human mind in an evolutionary perspective. Prominent representatives such as Cosmides, Tooby and Buss have proposed that a focus on man's evolutionary history of natural selection is the best way to unify psychology with hard science (foundational publications are Barkow *et al.*, 1992; Cosmides and Tooby, 1994; Buss, 1995). They assume that the invariant core of human nature has a genetic basis, but they do not come up with genetic analyses. Instead they reconstruct our past by an analysis of our present behaviours supplemented with conjectures about past behaviours. Evolutionary psychology has spawned evolutionary psychotherapy (Gilbert and Bailey, 2000), with evolutionary psychoanalysis as a special variant (Slavin and Kriegman, 1992), and evolutionary psychiatry (Stevens and Price, 1996; McGuire and Troisi, 1998), where the same kind of approach exists with an emphasis on maladaptive behaviour and mental illness. Here is an example. Stevens and Price (1996: 143) hypothesise that schizoid personalities have been an asset in ancestral human populations when groups had to split as resources became inadequate. Such personalities would have had the charisma needed to inspire the departing group with a sense of mission.

Research in these disciplines is speculative, as behaviour does not fossilise, and it often distorts evolutionary biology (for critical comments, see Davies, 1996; Griffiths, 1996; Richardson, 1996; Looren de Jong and Van der Steen, 1998; Lloyd, 1999; Rose and Rose, 2000; Van der Steen, 2000a). The philosopher of biology Brandon (1990) has demonstrated by a detailed analysis of a relatively simple case, heavy metal tolerance in plants, that reconstructions of evolutionary histories are hard to obtain. Non-biologists attempting to reconstruct the history of our mental make-up vastly underestimate the difficulties.

We do recognise the importance of evolutionary biology for medicine, but it lies elsewhere. Considering infectious diseases, for example, we need to know about short-term evolutionary processes that alter the behaviour of pathogens. Ewald (1994), in a groundbreaking book on evolutionary epidemiology, has rightly warned against the lack of evolutionary thinking in medicine's approach of infectious diseases, and Frank (2002), in a more recent book, has charted the relations between immunology and the evolution of pathogens, with far-reaching implications for the understanding and the treatment of infectious diseases (see also the comments on malaria in the main text). Nesse and Williams (1994 and 1998) have shown that evolutionary analyses illuminate many features of somatic disease. Here is an example. Bacteria need iron. Hence it is reasonable to assume that the reduction of blood iron after the invasion by pathogens is an evolved defence response. Physicians not trained in evolutionary thinking may not be aware of this and help the pathogen rather than the patient by prescribing iron. It is unfortunate that this kind of work gets little attention in mainstream medicine, whereas speculative evolutionary views of mental illness are gaining prominence.

The blood iron example illustrates the importance of functional analyses as a supplement of causal analyses. The evolved defence response has the function of protecting us against pathogens. Philosophers of biology have produced a large literature on biological functions (see for example Allen *et al.*, 1998; Buller, 1999), and for biologists functional thinking is an indispensable part of their trade. But medical professionals have only assimilated functional analysis to a limited extent. As genetics and molecular biology are getting more prominent roles in medicine, the importance of biological functions tends to recede farther to the background. To understand functions, we have to consider levels of organisation up to the level of the entire organism.

In the philosophy of biology, levels of organisation have always been an important subject, with the problem of reduction at centre stage. Should it be possible to reduce theories about high levels of organisation to low-level theories? The view that this kind of theory reduction is possible represents an old ideal. Nowadays, almost no philosopher of biology subscribes to it. If reduction is possible at all, it will have to be logically complex (see for example Bechtel and Richardson, 1993; Schaffner, 1993; Sarkar, 1998). A pronounced emphasis on genetics in biomedical research does not sit well with this complexity.

Simplistic views of the causal roles of genes in organisms result also from a negligence of developmental biology in much theorising. Evolutionary biology and genetics associated with it have progressed in disregard of developmental biology. In the philosophy of biology, a group of researchers has forged a synthesis called developmental systems theory (Oyama *et al.*, 2001). Other researchers from a variety of disciplines have also emphasised the need of putting genetics in the context of development (Raff, 1996; Elman *et al.*, 1997; Schlichting and Pigliucci, 1998; Van der Weele, 1999; Lagercrantz *et al.*, 2002; see also Sterelny and Griffiths, 1999, who present an excellent overview of philosophy of biology). These researchers emphasise the continual interaction of genes and environmental factors during development. The interaction is a two-way process in which genetic factors are by no means a constant element. The idea that our genetic endowment is a kind of program that generates adult features is a grave mistake. It is true that some relatively stable developmental configurations exist, which admit of the metaphor that particular genes "code" for a particular disease. But in most situations this metaphor is dangerously misleading.

In a different context, genetic engineering and biotechnology, Ho (1998) has a similar message. She argues that modern genetics feeding large industrial enterprises is scientifically flawed. The idea that we can insert genes coding for desirable features in the genetic program of organisms, and end up with new organisms with a predictable overall make-up, is utterly naive. To some extent it works in occasional cases, but the inherent dangers in the form of unexpected side effects are legion, in genetics applied to medicine and in genetics applied to agriculture (for critical analyses of genetic engineering in agriculture, see also Lappé and Bailey, 1999; Charles, 2001). Genetics is over-dominant in biomedical research into disease. That is why we search in our book for environmental compensation.

We do not think that integrative super-theories of disease are feasible. Instead we have to draw on miscellaneous theories, each with strengths and weaknesses. We side here with the philosopher of biology Keller (2002) who in a different context, that of biological development, concludes that we have to live with a plurality of explanatory styles:

> The central concern of this book has been with the de facto multiplicity of explanatory styles in scientific practice, reflecting the manifest diversity of epistemological goals which researchers bring to their task. But I also want to argue that the investigation of processes as inherently complex as biological

> development may in fact require such diversity. Explanatory pluralism, I suggest, is now not simply a reflection of differences in epistemological cultures but a positive virtue in itself, representing our best chance of coming to terms with the world around us. (Keller, 2002: 300)

Chapter 2

The Spectrum of Diseases

2.1. Introduction

Nowadays, *drapetomania* does not ring a bell for most people. It did in the nineteenth century, at least in the United States. Official Western medicine then recognised drapetomania, the tendency of slaves to run away from their owners, as a disease that commonly afflicted black persons.

Being civilised, you may feel that this kind of oddity has no foothold any more in our culture, since modern medicine and psychiatry, based as they are on objective science, have outgrown old shortcomings and superstitions. We are not pessimists, but we would not be quite ready to share this optimistic feeling. With hindsight, drapetomania is easily dismissed as a harmful fabrication of fictitious disease, in a culture violating human rights. Less easy is it to recognise harmful fabrications of our own era for what they are.

Are you sure that medicine and psychiatry are on the right track, morally and scientifically, in providing millions of persons with drugs after having diagnosed them as being depressed in some medical sense? It does not make sense to us that so many persons should suffer from any such disease. We rather see much unhappiness arising from adverse social conditions in our culture. Indeed, some drugs targeted at unhappiness construed as disease may self-fulfillingly transform it into real disease.

Diabetes is a disease, a collection of several diseases actually. The common cold, influenza, is a disease. Drapetomania is not a disease. Depression is a problem case. Perhaps the medical community mistakenly regards it as a disease. Or perhaps depression is a proper disease label for limited numbers of persons, the label being overblown, mistakenly to fit healthy persons in unhealthy situations. We anyhow do not believe that the professionals are entirely right.

The bone of contention is here that some would place particular conditions inside the *category* of disease, whereas others would put them outside it. To decide the issue, we need proper definitions for words such as “disease” and “health.” Such definitions must not be confused with definitions for particular diseases such as diabetes. The fact that we can define “diabetes” by no means implies that we can define “disease.”

Philosophers of medicine have written much about disease, the category. The book *What is disease?* (Humber and Almeder, 1997) portrays the most representative philosophical views. It contains chapters by eight well-known authors with expertise in the philosophy of medicine. The authors answer the title question in very different ways.

The most significant issue for the authors concerns values. Some argue that disease is a category with specimens studied by medical science in a value-free manner. Others hold that the notion of disease is linked with human values. The two views, which come in many varieties, are known as naturalism and normativism, respectively. Naturalists and normativists agree that we need value-laden words to connote the patient’s perspective. They mostly use the word “illness” with this connotation. The disagreement is over “disease.” Naturalists want to have some such word to cover diseases in an objective, scientific way. Normativists claim that such a thing is impossible since values cannot be divorced from the core of medicine.

Disputes about this have been going on for a long time, and they do not show signs of termination by resolution. As we do not wish to partake of such disputes, we use here words such as “disease” without defining them. Intended meanings have to be clear from the context. Part of the problem is presumably that the words have different meanings in different contexts, so that the search for a single definition is misguided. This is not to deny that decisions concerning the disease status of problem cases such as depression are important. They clearly are. Neither would we deny that the issue of human values in medicine is important. It clearly is. But the fabrication of some overarching definition of “disease” is apparently not a fruitful way to address these things.

Textbooks of medicine seldom offer definitions or discussions of the general categories of disease and illness, and others such as disorder, syndrome, malady and injury. To understand how they deal with the categories, we have to look at how they deal with particular cases. We are going to look at a sample of cases in a critical, analytical way. After some general considerations in Section 2, we discuss in Section 3 muscle diseases, fibromyalgia, the chronic fatigue syndrome and rheumatoid arthritis, in this order. We do not describe these diseases in great detail. Instead, we analyse representative passages from the medical literature. The analyses uncover presuppositions in medical thinking which are easily overlooked. As well, they reveal elements of arbitrariness in the characterisation and the classification of diseases. The arbitrariness as such is not a bad thing; it is unavoidable as nature is not fully geared to human purposes. But if we fail to recognise arbitrariness for what it is, we run the risk that we distort realities of disease, at worst by creating modern variants of drapetomania.

2.2. Diseases, Symptoms, and Signs

An introduction to the symptoms and signs of clinical medicine (Gray and Toghill, 2001), written for clinical students during their early days on the wards, is a good source to start with. The two key terms in the title refer to different aspects of diseases. Doctors generally use the term "symptoms" for features experienced by the patient, and reserve the term "signs" for underlying features revealed by medical examination.

When a clinician or a clinical student meets a patient for the first time, they need to investigate what is wrong with him or her. This is done by history taking and clinical examination. The first part of the book, written by the editors, is devoted to these activities. We quote from the beginning of the first chapter, which concerns history taking:

> Each disease tends to present in a fairly characteristic way. Doctors try to tie together the symptoms a patient reports, the signs of bodily change seen on clinical examination and the physiological and pathological changes found in various blood and other tests into a recognizable pattern typical of a specific disease. Having thus made a *diagnosis*, the doctor, drawing on experience and knowledge, can discuss with the patient the expected *prognosis* and the range of options for treatment. ... The most important part of the whole process is 'taking a history'. ... A history is a detailed account of the patient's current illness; significant factors which might predispose to illness, details of any previous medical history; current and previous drug treatment; any relevant history of familial illnesses; and personal and social history and habits. ... For some diseases like migraine, there are no helpful investigations, so the diagnosis rests solely on a well-taken history. (Gray and Toghill, 2001: 3)

This passage, like the rest of the book, is well written and to the point. We would not criticise the text as such, but we have critical comments that come to mind once we put it in broader contexts.

The meaning of the general term "disease," as in most other textbooks of medicine, is nowhere clarified in the book. Yet, some understanding of "disease" must be presupposed. Consider the first sentence: "Each disease tends to present in a fairly characteristic way." This is in effect a strong claim about "disease," the general category compounded of particular diseases. The authors presuppose here that the reader understands the notion of disease. Let us take this for granted in considering the claim. If reasons existed to regard the claim as problematic because the notion is unclear, they would not be a fitting subject for inexperienced clinical students. The students need some certainties and routines to begin with. In different contexts, though, doubts concerning the claim would be a natural thing.

Should the claim be regarded as acceptable? Our response to this question may surprise you. Even if we had detailed knowledge concerning all domains of medicine, we would not feel able to pass judgment on the claim. That is because it can be understood in different ways. We have to understand what it means before deciding whether it is acceptable, and that is possible only with prior understanding concerning the meaning of "disease."

Conceivably, medical professionals could decide to reserve the term "disease" for items that "present in a fairly characteristic way." If they did that, then you would not have a disease if the doctor did not find a characteristic presentation, or you would have a disease with characteristics that will develop later on, or you would have a rare disease so that the doctor forgivably misses the presentation. Remarkably, from this interpretation the claim we are considering would be true *by definition*. It would not represent any facts. This would make disputes about the acceptability of the claim superfluous, because the issue thus reduces to mere terminology.

Another potential problem with the claim concerns classification. The claim appears to presuppose that diseases are discrete items assignable to the general category of "disease." Instances of a particular disease should normally present its characteristic features (symptoms, signs), and different diseases should have different features associated with them, of course with possible overlaps.

However, things cannot be that simple. Suppose, you get "the flu" and that you are unfortunate as a pneumonia ensues from it which happens to resist the antibiotics you receive, after which your condition deteriorates so much that you are plagued by hallucinations and delusions. We could describe the course of these events as a succession of three different diseases, "the flu," pneumonia and psychosis. But we may also choose to describe all this as a single disease, severe pneumonia caused by an infection with a particular strain of bacteria, with hallucinations and delusions as symptoms of severity. The choice to be made is somewhat arbitrary in this situation.

The decision to adopt a particular classification does affect the claim we are considering ("Each disease tends to present in a fairly characteristic way"). The "characteristic ways" of diseases cannot simply be patterns existing "out there" in nature apart from our theorising. The patterns are of our own making, however well they may fit phenomena we *choose* to focus on. Nature does not provide us with diseases as neatly ordered packages. But medical professionals have to use routines that presuppose that neatly ordered packages exist. It is like they have to adopt an enforced make-believe with roots in reality that vary in strength, depending on circumstances created by nature and by ourselves.

Classifications deserve special scrutiny whenever patients can have more than one disease, a phenomenon known as comorbidity. If comorbidities are common in a particular disease, this may well represent artificiality of classification. In some instances, comorbidity may be a sign that a classification has outrun its usefulness (see for example Chapter 6).

Back to the passage quoted; we are finished with the first sentence. In accordance with common views, the passage makes clear that medicine, in diagnoses, ultimately aims to conceptualise diseases as somatic phenomena (cf. "bodily change," "physiological and pathological changes," and so forth). Nothing is wrong with this in itself, because medical professionals, like the rest of us, have to confine work and expertise to particular areas. But human beings are not mere physical bodies. Mental processes belong with diseases as well as physical processes in bodies. A medical focus on the body alone may thus be inadequate in some circumstances, theoretically and practically.

The emphasis on the body does characterise medicine's notion of disease and the framing of diagnoses, once reached. But, as the passage quoted indicates, the context must also be considered. The symptoms reported by the patient (to be distinguished from signs) include psychological and social matters in addition to problems with their bodies. Case histories (cf. "taking a history") similarly have a broad scope. The description in the passage represents a characteristic trend in medicine. The things mentioned (account of illness, factors which might predispose to illness, previous medical history, drug treatment, personal and social history and habits) refer to medical matters narrowly conceived (emphasis on the body), but also to psychosocial matters. The entire chapter from which the passage quoted was taken, suggests that this is a fundamental distinction.

Undue emphasis on the body may lead to a one-sided view of

illness. The distinction made here is a source of additional one-sidedness. It represents an incomplete classification of aetiological factors (factors causing disease). If biological factors are equated with factors concerning the body, and psychological factors are taken to represent environmental factors, we face a lacuna (see Van der Steen and Thung, 1988; Van der Steen, 1993b). We actually have here two classifications: internal *versus* external factors, and biological *versus* psychosocial factors. If we amalgamate them, we are missing internal psychological factors such as emotions, and external biological factors. This incompleteness, particularly negligence of the external biological environment, may cause a strong bias in medicine (for case studies, see for example Chapters 3 and 7).

Taking an adequate history is difficult in view of this potential bias. Researchers and clinicians anyhow face the problem that numerous causal factors play a role in any disease. It is inconceivable that they would be able to consider them all. They cannot do their work without a restrictive focus. This is appropriate, but when a focus becomes pervasively restrictive by an emphasis on particular causal factors, we may get undesirable situations (for case studies, see Chapters 3, 5, 7, 8 and 10). The one-sidedness mentioned would be an example of this.

This concludes our illustrations of elementary textbook medicine. Our reflective analysis indicates that seemingly simple ideas concerning disease may have an undercover of difficult, fundamental problems. The next section applies this kind of analysis to a more advanced level of medicine.

2.3. Deliveries of Advanced Medicine

Fatigue has recently become a plague. Conditions that go by names such as chronic fatigue syndrome and fibromyalgia are common. Unfortunately, medical professionals hardly know how to deal with them. Patients with the fatigue feel that something is wrong with their muscles. But the professionals have not found fault with the muscles. We analyse some existing views of elusive fatigue in this section, but we begin with "genuine" muscle diseases.

A chapter by Brooke (2001) in an advanced level text, *Disorders of voluntary muscle*, reviews the classification of muscle diseases. These diseases come in many kinds, but all of them show deteriorations of muscle function or morphology, seriously so in many cases. Brooke is concerned with "muscle diseases" in a narrow sense, with the primary pathology residing in the muscles themselves; he is not explicit about this, but the context makes it clear. He notes that muscle diseases have been classified for more than a century by their clinical appearance. But the old classification has been demolished by discoveries since the mid-1980s. Here is what Brooke (2001) has to say about the current situation:

> Patients with identical histories and findings have totally different genetic abnormalities. Patients with the same molecular defect appear radically different. It is enough to make the great clinicians turn in their grave and the diagnosticians slink back to their lairs. (...) [Many genetic abnormalities were discovered.]
>
> Patients were often detoured from the muscle clinic and sent for DNA studies before the examining physician had a chance to ply his trade. (...)
>
> At the start of the 1990s, I would have confidently predicted that the next long-lasting classification of muscle disease would be based on genetic abnormalities. This is no longer tenable and it is now apparent that any future classification will have to be based on the molecular abnormalities themselves. This should, in fact, have been self-evident. Except for the muscle diseases that are caused by remote factors such as vascular insufficiency or immunological attack, the root cause has to be an abnormality in the component mechanisms of the muscle 'machine.' These are all proteins, each of which may be governed by one or several genes. We should turn our attention to these proteins and assemble them into some order. (Brooke, 2001: 374)

Brooke subsequently presents the outlines of the new classification in the making. Names of old diseases are now replaced by names that refer to deficiencies in proteins associated with various anatomical components of muscles.

Brooke's formulations suggest that the new classification represents findings wrestled from nature by new sophisticated research. But we should not forget that the new system is also a matter of *decision*. An alternative option would be to retain old ways and to stipulate that, in decisions concerning classifications, homogeneity of symptoms among patients should outrank homogeneity of protein abnormalities among patients. That would result in diseases that are heterogeneous with respect to genetic abnormalities and protein abnormalities. Or we could make genetic abnormalities the prime criterion of classification and pay the price that this would generate diseases that are heterogeneous with respect to protein abnormalities and symptoms.

One phrasing in the passage quoted is particularly fascinating: The root cause has to be an abnormality in the component mechanisms of the muscle "machine." What should "root cause" be taken to mean? We assume that Brooke presupposes here that, if symptoms of a disease result from a malfunctioning organ, then abnormal features of the organ should be regarded as the most significant causes—"root causes"—of the disease. Thus, he would allot a subordinate role to other causal factors, for example genetic factors underlying the abnormal features, or environmental factors influencing the expression of the genetic factors. This could mean that Brooke would *define* "root cause" in this way. But from this interpretation, his argument that muscle diseases must be classified by reference to the abnormal features of the organ *because* they represent root causes, is somewhat misleading. The clause "because they represent root causes" would not provide additional information in this case, as it would be true by definition. Our reflections on the passage quoted anyhow illustrate that classifications reflect choices made by us in addition to facts of nature.

Muscle diseases are mostly rare. Fibromyalgia and the chronic fatigue syndrome (CFS), diseases with muscle problems, not muscle diseases in a strict sense, are common. Both are syndromes. Medical professionals use this term in preference to "disease" when they are dealing with a cluster of symptoms without known cause. The term "disorder" is also used in this situation. Fibromyalgia and CFS have both been attributed to many different factors, but consistent evidence in favour of any particular factor has not been obtained (for surveys of research and representative views, see Pillemer, 1994; Chalmers *et al.*, 1995; Russell, 1996; Skelly and Helm, 1999; Campling and Sharpe, 2000; Moss-Morris and Petrie, 2000; Duncan, 2001, Bennett, 2002).

We examine a chapter by Kissel and Miller (1999) on the two syndromes, from another book on muscle diseases, *Muscle diseases, blue books in practical neurology, vol. 2*. Their text is a representative illustration of how medicine approaches elusive illnesses.

Muscle pain and fatigue are common. According to some population studies, as many as 20 per cent of individuals reported muscle pain or discomfort. The symptoms are often frustrating for clinician and patient alike, because diagnosis is difficult. They may be due to a wide variety of general medical, rheumatological, orthopaedic, neurological, or psychiatric conditions. If prolonged evaluations of patients do not uncover any of these conditions, we are left with a diagnosis of fibromyalgia or chronic fatigue syndrome. We discuss fibromyalgia first.

Kissel and Miller report that fibromyalgia is the most common cause of muscle aches and pains in the general population; some studies indicate that about 2 per cent of individuals fulfil diagnostic criteria for the syndrome. As yet, we have no therapies which are generally successful.

Upon exclusion of other known diseases, current diagnostic criteria for fibromyalgia include two major criteria: widespread diffuse muscle pain for at least 3 months, and the presence of so-called tender points in at least 11 of 18 defined sites. These points hurt upon being touched. The criteria help medical professionals choose a diagnostic label for patients, but they are somewhat arbitrary. It is implausible that 3 months and 11 sites instead of, say, 5 months and 13 sites, should represent "natural" features of a disorder.

In the previous section, we argued that nature does not provide us with diseases as neat packages. All classifications of diseases are arbitrary and artificial to some extent, even though the diseases are rooted in reality. Some entities recognised as diseases are distinct and have strong roots. Fibromyalgia has weak roots at best. It is to a great extent an entity of our own making.

Kissel and Miller (1999) note that fibromyalgia is controversial:

> Some investigators feel that fibromyalgia does not exist as a definable entity, while others believe it is a strictly psychogenic phenomenon ... . Still others have hypothesized that fibromyalgia, while a distinct entity, does not fit into a traditional biomedical model of disease and is best considered in a psychosocial conceptualisation ... . Despite continuing controversy, the vast majority of clinicians and investigators ... has embraced fibromyalgia as a valid syndrome that is as real as any other condition (e.g., migraine headaches) for which the diagnostic criteria are predominantly clinical and the underlying pathophysiology poorly understood. ... From a practical perspective, because the concept of fibromyalgia has been embraced by the vast majority of clinicians, it does no good for the neuromuscular practitioner to deny that it exists ... . (Kissel and Miller, 1999: 41)

Several themes in this passage merit reflection. To start with, fibromyalgia has us ponder over roles of biological and psychological or psychosocial factors in medicine. In the most common view, medical theory should be concerned only with biology. Psychology has its place in medical practice, but it has no role to play in medical theories.

This view is known as the biomedical model (in a narrow sense of the term not embraced by all researchers). It presupposes that biological and psychological processes can be kept apart in theory if not in practice. The presupposition represents a fundamental philosophy that many, including ourselves, would reject. Common sense alone suggests that we should not take it for granted.

Consider the term "psychogenic." What meaning could it have here? The following hypothetical example illustrates that we have a problem on our hands. A particular person is chronically sad because a partner is terminally ill, and gets a heart attack after a long period of sadness. For the sake of argument, we disregard the role of predisposing factors. If the sadness caused the heart attack in that the attack would not have occurred without it, would that imply that the attack was psychogenic? In a certain sense this may be so, but the technical label of "psychogenic" would be misleading because being sad cannot be *merely* psychological. Emotions always affect the body, and we could as well stipulate that the heart attack was somatogenic as physiological processes accompanying the sadness must have caused it.

In the case of fibromyalgia, no consensus exists about antecedent biological aspects. But such aspects should exist, and antecedent psychological aspects should also exist. This is not to say that all the antecedents, once known, have to be regarded as aetiologically significant causes. Decisions concerning the significance of biological or psychological factors are best postponed until particular factors are known in the first place. We are belabouring this point, because patients who have symptoms without *known* underlying organic aspects, run the risk of simply getting the advice "Go see a psychiatrist." If such a thing happened to us, we would get mad.

Crucial in the passage quoted are the terms "valid" and "real." We object to the use of the term "validity" in this context (see also Chapter 6, with a similar comment on "schizophrenia"). To be acceptable, diagnoses in medicine have to meet the requirements of reliability and validity. A judgment is reliable if professionals agree about it, whereas it is valid if it represents things as they are. If the majority of clinicians and investigators have indeed "embraced fibromyalgia," and if they use the notion of fibromyalgia in the same way, then a reliable diagnosis exists. But to be valid, a diagnosis must offer more than mere terminological agreement about symptoms. It must be embedded in some theory and preferably have predictive value. That is not so for fibromyalgia. We have patients with particular, loosely defined symptoms without a scientific explanation. And we have invented a name for the symptoms. *That is all.*

The term "real" is also misleading. Medical professionals who adopt the diagnosis of fibromyalgia as "real," do two things: They accept a definition, and they assume that the definition applies to some existing persons. Again, *that is all.* To be "real" in the sense of representing a bona fide disease, a diagnosis should also be valid.

We wonder what the last sentence in the passage quoted means. "It does no good ... to deny that it exists." Should this be taken to mean that the nature of fibromyalgia has to be determined by majority vote? If so, then we can but comment that we wish to vote in accordance with our own conscience.

Kissel and Miller state that all sorts of laboratory investigations concerning fibromyalgia have failed to uncover abnormalities. From this, they infer the conclusion that fibromyalgia is not a genuine muscle disease, since no muscle abnormalities have been found. From published studies, Kissel and Miller (1999) infer two additional, remarkable conclusions:

> The second conclusion is that fibromyalgia is probably not a single disease, but rather a chronic pain syndrome that overlaps with other similar conditions, such as chronic fatigue syndrome ..., irritable bowel syndrome, migraine headaches, and various psychiatric disorders ... . This concept leads immediately to the third conclusion: It is extremely unlikely that a single definable cause for fibromyalgia will be found. (...) Much current attention has therefore turned to a psychosocial model of fibromyalgia, focusing on the concept that the pain of fibromyalgia may represent up-regulation of abnormal central pain mechanisms, which may result from a number of genetic, biochemical, infectious, or traumatic events ... . According to this model, fibromyalgia results from a generalized pain intolerance that is due to functional abnormalities in the central nervous system. [Some studies appear to support this.] (Kissel and Miller, 1999: 45)

This passage baffles us. A passage preceding this one, which we quoted, stipulates that "the vast majority of clinicians and investigators ... has embraced fibromyalgia as a valid syndrome that is as real as any other condition." We objected that this use of the terms "valid" and "real" is misplaced, as it represents mere consensus about terminology and definition. Our objection is now being confirmed. If fibromyalgia overlaps with other syndromes, and if reasons exist to assume that it is not a single disease, then the majority of clinicians and investigators is indeed embracing a fictitious entity. Let us be frank, then, and admit that the diagnosis is at most a pragmatic label attached to patients, to be used when authorities, or colleagues, or patients themselves, insist that they want a label.

The passage quoted also calls for comments on biological *versus* psychosocial factors. On the one hand, the message seems to be that various biological factors may be causal antecedents of fibromyalgia, and that as yet unknown abnormalities in the central nervous system may explain the pain symptoms. That would concur with the biomedical model. On the other hand, we are told that fibromyalgia invites a psychosocial model. How can that be? The crucial term here is "functional." Medical professionals often use this term for syndromes with unknown organic causes. This usage easily invites the fallacy that psychosocial factors must be significant if we cannot find significant biological factors (cf. our earlier comments on the term "psychogenic").

Kissel and Miller (1999: 46) report that several studies have documented a high comorbidity (20 per cent) of fibromyalgia and psychiatric disorders, especially depression. That should not surprise us. Chronic pain easily provokes feelings of depression. Furthermore, doctors who provide the patient with a "psychosocial" diagnosis may contribute to such feelings.

Kissel and Miller also present an overview of the chronic fatigue syndrome (CFS), which is mostly characterised by fatigue over many years after a sudden onset. Their approach of the CFS resembles that of fibromyalgia, and we would have similar comments. Therefore we do not discuss their view of CFS. Instead, we briefly summarise a theoretical investigation of the syndrome by one of us (Van der Steen, 2000b).

The idea that CFS is a mystery, is common. I (WJS) decided to test common knowledge by a search of the medical literature. Soon I found out that, overall, articles explicitly dealing with CFS indicate that we know next to nothing about aetiology and possible treatments. But literature on muscle fatigue in general provided some interesting cues. Here is what I uncovered.

Muscle fatigue is a characteristic feature in patients suffering from enzyme deficiencies, in particular acyl CoA (co-enzyme A) dehydrogenase deficiency, myoadenylate deaminase deficiency, and many types of glycogenoses. Handbooks about such deficiencies report that patients have very serious symptoms, in addition to muscle fatigue and other symptoms that are common in CFS. But a thorough search of primary sources (research articles) revealed that for almost all the deficiencies, patients are known who do not have the nasty symptoms, but only symptoms as found in CFS. If their deficiency had not been known, these patients would probably have received the diagnosis of CFS.

Inquiries among specialists and patients showed that few of them know about this. That is deplorable because a minority of so-called CFS-patients could benefit from a known treatment: Some of the patients who have an acyl CoA dehydrogenase deficiency, benefit from a simple treatment with vitamin B2.

The lacuna I uncovered should have been spotted years ago. Super-specialisation in medicine combined with a huge and ever increasing research output has obviously prevented this. Also, medical professionals may have a tendency to underrate biological variability and so miss non-standard explanations.

CFS is presumably a heterogeneous syndrome. Hence, my enzyme hypothesis may only apply to few CFS patients. I do know that at least one patient recovered after a vitamin B2 therapy, undertaken on the advice of a physician who read my article.

The two cases considered so far, "genuine" muscle disorders linked with abnormal proteins in the muscles themselves, and muscle pain and fatigue without known cause, are extremes at opposite sides of a continuum. Let us see what we learn from a comparison of the extremes.

The opening claim of the passage quoted in the previous section provides a useful starting point for the comparison. "Each disease tends to present in a fairly characteristic way." We commented that the claim is unclear. From one interpretation, it expresses a definitional truth: If the notion of disease is reserved for entities with a characteristic presentation, then the claim is true in a trivial way as it expresses something about word usage rather than revealing insights concerning diseases. The example of fibromyalgia shows that we face here a genuine puzzle. Fibromyalgia does not have a characteristic presentation in the sense intended in this passage, and it is controversial with respect to disease status. If we denied syndromes such as fibromyalgia disease status for lack of a characteristic presentation, then the claim would become a definitional truth.

We also argued that the claim appears to presuppose the existence of a well-ordered natural classification. That is problematic, since classifications are often arbitrary and artificial; comorbidities may thus result from inadequate classifications. The examples in the present section appear to confirm this.

The claim may also be misleading for the following reason. It could invite the inference that, if most diseases have characteristic presentations, then most persons with a disease must also have a characteristic presentation. That would be a fallacy. Suppose that we accept fibromyalgia as a bona fide disease that happens to be a rare exception to the claim because it has no clear presentation. The muscle diseases discussed by Brooke, which come in many different kinds, do have clear presentations. These diseases are all rare, whereas fibromyalgia is common. We have here a situation in which most diseases have a clear presentation, whereas most patients happen to suffer from a disease without a clear presentation. The thesis that most diseases have characteristic presentations is therefore compatible with the thesis that most individual patients may not show characteristic presentations at all. The point is worth making to avoid bias that puts patients suffering from disorders such as fibromyalgia at a disadvantage.

Muscle disorders, according to Brooke, all have a "root cause" (a notion we criticised), namely an abnormal protein located at specific sites in muscles. Fibromyalgia has no known causes. Rheumatoid arthritis, our next example, represents yet another situation. Much remains to be discovered concerning its aetiology and pathology, but the existing evidence indicates that it involves many causal factors, none of them deserving a label such as "root cause." We give a brief description based on a textbook by Jennekens and Kater, *Neurology of the inflammatory connective tissue diseases* (1999, Chapter 9).

Rheumatoid arthritis is common: It affects about 1 per cent of the world population. It is one of the inflammatory connective tissue diseases, which belong to the so-called autoimmune disorders. In these disorders, the immune system, normally a defence system, attacks components of the body itself. Rheumatoid arthritis is characterised by an inflammation of joints, particularly of hands and feet, and also blood vessels. Secondarily, serious disfigurement involving bone and muscle loss may occur. If the spine is affected, neurological symptoms may develop on top of this. Usually, the disease is slowly progressive. It may in the end be invalidating and it tends to shorten life span.

Researchers assume that some environmental agent, possibly a microorganism, triggers the autoimmune response. But the predisposition of susceptible individuals also plays a role. Once the inflammatory response is set in motion, numerous causal factors in the body contribute to disease progression.

Let us compare this disease with muscle diseases. Any of them, like rheumatoid arthritis, may exhibit severe symptoms ultimately affecting many organs. But the muscle diseases have a different aetiology, with a salient role for genetic factors affecting vital proteins rather than environmental triggers impairing the immune system (unknown factors in the case of rheumatoid arthritis). Also, pathological processes in the body are less "diffuse" in muscle diseases than in rheumatoid arthritis.

Should we expect that more research will ultimately unravel remaining mysteries of rheumatoid arthritis—and all the persistent mysteries of fibromyalgia? Will we manage to identify "root causes" also for these diseases, or disease conglomerates? We have doubts, though we would not deny that progress is possible in the way of discovering additional factors in the causation and the progression of disease, perhaps even successful therapies—which are sorely needed for all the diseases we reviewed.

Our doubts concern the common optimistic idea that modern biomedical research is able in principle to arrive at "the" ultimate truth about the causes of all diseases. In passing, we have mentioned several reasons for tempering this kind of optimism. We list them here with some additional comments.

- Classifications are always arbitrary to some extent, the degree of arbitrariness depending among other things on the degree of natural order that happens to be present in the case at hand. Owing to biological variability, any clustering of features generating allegedly distinct diseases will also generate exceptions and overlaps.

- Genetic factors and environmental factors interact in many ways, and their effects change in the course of development. In all diseases, numerous factors interact. If we are lucky, we come across a disease in which one or a few factors have effects so salient, that we are justified to see it as a distinct entity admitting of an unambiguous description. No reason exists to assume that nature has a tendency to make this kind of luck pervasive.

- Research concerning diseases, like all research, is necessarily selective. Selectivity is a potential source of undesirable bias. The example of the chronic fatigue syndrome indicates that selectivity may even make us miss important ideas within a narrowly defined specialism. Undesirable forms of bias exist also at the level of entire disciplines. We briefly mentioned one example, the common trend in medicine to equate biological factors with internal factors, and psychosocial factors with external factors. External biological factors in the domain of ecology may thus fall by the wayside. The role of diet in health and disease is an important example of this. Ecologists would be aware that diet may have a profound influence on health and disease. Medical professionals know about this, of course, but the role of diet is

> undervalued in much medicine. It so happens that rheumatoid arthritis is presumably a paradigm of diseases fostered by dietary deficiencies (see Chapter 8). Yet mainstream medicine ignores this.

We do hope that biased selectivity in research will become an important theme in medical writings. Overt disclosure of selectivity should be the first step toward decreasing its impact.

2.4. Conclusions

1. The general notion of disease is elusive since the category of diseases is heterogeneous. This may invite the mistake of seeing disease where none exists. The labelling of ordinary human suffering as depression in a medical sense would be an example.

2. Classifications and characterisations of diseases are to some extent arbitrary. Diseases are in part facts of nature, in part our invention. For example, medical professionals nowadays tend to characterise muscle diseases by protein abnormalities in muscles. This may be useful theoretically and practically, but nature does not quite dictate such a thing.

3. The biomedical model invites a fallacious tendency to regard diseases with unknown somatic causes such as fibromyalgia and the chronic fatigue syndrome as "psychogenic."

4. One-sided research may prevent the discovery of somatic causes of disease. The possibility that an enzyme deficiency may explain some cases of the chronic fatigue syndrome is an example of this.

5. Ecology deserves more attention in medicine. The study of environmental causes of disease is often restricted to the psychosocial factors, in disregard of ecology. The existing emphasis in biomedical research on genetics and molecular biology also detracts from ecology.

Chapter 3

Diseases, Causes, and Treatments: New Vistas

3.1. Introduction

Ideal medications would be like magic bullets that cure disease in a short time without side effects. Such magic bullets are rare if they exist at all, but medicine at times comes close to the ideal. Drug treatments of "gastric ulcer" (ulcers of the stomach or the adjacent part of the gut, the duodenum) look like a near hit. Nowadays, drugs often cure the ulcers in a short time, not entirely without side effects and other disadvantages, though. The drugs are not our concern here; they are discussed in Chapter 8. Instead we look back in time at fates of persons who had ulcers prior to the advent of the drugs.

The older among us may remember that, a few decades ago, ulcer disease called for much rest, a cautious way of life, and considerable restrictions on food and beverages. The idea was then that stress is the culprit causing the disease, and that long lasting avoidance of stress combined with moderation is the best remedy. The identification of the bacterium *Helicobacter pylori* as the "real" culprit set in motion the development of new, successful drug treatments (for details and critical comments, see Chapters 8 and 9).

The more remote past has a surprise in store for us. Many persons have been cured from ulcers by a simple treatment with honey (Root-Bernstein and Root-Bernstein, 1997: 38-40). Physicians in the Arabic world, the Caucasus and Russia have for centuries treated the ulcers successfully with this innocuous substance. With the benefit of hindsight, we can explain this in a satisfactory way. Concentrated doses of honey taken orally appear to kill *H. pylori.* Honey presumably exerts its antibiotic effect by stimulating white blood cells to destroy the bacteria, and by creating a chemical environment in which the bacteria cannot survive. Furthermore, honey contains active substances with antiseptic properties. We have here an unpleasant disease that can be cured by a harmless effective treatment. The treatment has been known for centuries, but it has been debarred from modern medicine.

In their fascinating book, *Honey, mud, maggots, and other*

medical marvels: the science behind folk remedies and old wives' tales, Root-Bernstein and Root-Bernstein (1997) provide many more examples of useful remedies from medicine's past and from folk medicine. For example, upon proper precautions, *maggots* are an excellent remedy for nasty, festering wounds. The maggots eat away rotten cells and so help cure infections. Doctors or patients may understandably opt, though, for a different treatment on the ground that they do not like the sight of the maggots.

In the last chapter of their book, the authors analyse some factors that hamper an optimal usage of folk wisdom in official medicine. The treatments are often cheap, and they represent knowledge that cannot be patented. Pharmaceutical industries therefore have no incentive to develop them for the market. New treatments must pass approval by regulatory bodies that demand proof by expensive tests. This is an economic hurdle which many folk remedies cannot pass. Failing economic support, medicine may thus ignore potentially valuable treatments (see also the volume edited by Brady, 2001, which analyses connections between conventional medicine and folk medicine in the United States, and contains an extensive bibliography).

The choice of treatments to be included in official medicine is obviously selective owing to cultural factors. In the previous chapter, we argued that selectivity exists also for theoretical reasons. It is impossible, for example, that medical professionals consider all causal antecedents of a disease. They have to be selective in the choice of factors to be regarded as significant causes. Selectivity as such is not a bad thing, but persistent selectivity may create undesirable bias.

In the present chapter we argue that particular effects of the environment—biological, social and political—on health and disease do not receive the attention they deserve. This is an example of bias with far-reaching implications.

3.2. Evolution, Food, and Affluence

The honey example in the Introduction is from recent history. The more remote past has also much to tell us about health and disease. To illustrate this, we summarise an article by Eaton and Konner (1985) that provides a reconstruction of diets of our Palaeolithic ancestors, which comes close to the optimal present-day diet. The article is based on a wealth of evidence from evolutionary biology and several other disciplines (for additional comments and more recent sources, see Chapter 7.4).

Our genetic constitution cannot have changed much since truly modern human beings, *Homo sapiens sapiens*, appeared on the scene, about 40,000 years ago. Eaton and Konner argue that our dietary flexibility is high, but that modern diets have moved beyond the range that fits the genetic constitution of our ancestors and ourselves. Dietary habits adopted over the past 100 years contribute to diseases of affluence such as coronary heart disease, hypertension, diabetes and cancers. These diseases are virtually unknown in surviving hunter-gatherer populations whose lifestyles resemble those of preagricultural human beings.

Common wisdom has it that such diseases are a by-product of long life spans. The assumption is here that natural selection does not eliminate diseases of old age, since they do not diminish reproductive success. But this cannot be the whole story, as young people in the West have asymptomatic forms of these diseases, whereas old persons in "primitive" cultures are free of them.

Diets have varied with times and places, but one thing is clear. Our preagicultural ancestors often consumed much meat from game (see also Stanford, 1999) or fish. The fact that humans who relied predominantly on agriculture were shorter than ancestors or descendants of them who consumed much animal protein, suggests that their diet was suboptimal. Our body length has recently increased again. We obviously make the most of our food with respect to conversion into body mass. But the quality of our diet is so far from optimal that it causes much chronic disease.

Our domestic livestock contains much smaller quantities of polyunsaturated fatty acids (PUFAs) than wild game. The so-called omega-3 PUFAs are particularly important. Diets in "civilised" countries fall far short of meeting our physiological requirements of these PUFAs. Omega-3 PUFAs benefit our health in many ways. They have antiatherosclerotic properties, for example. No wonder then, that atherosclerosis is common in our culture (for details, see Chapter 7).

Our plant food also deviates considerably from natural diets. It does not contain adequate amounts of omega-3 PUFAs and other important nutrients. Foragers hardly consume small cereal grains, which have become staples for "civilised" people. They relied on roots, beans, nuts, tubers and fruits.

Eaton and Conner suggest that we change our diets accordingly. Evidence is accumulating that current diets impair our health. Official dietary recommendations are considerably at variance with their suggestions (for references, see Chapter 7). Disturbingly, their insights are disregarded in many areas of medicine in spite of their being based on reliable literature that spans half a century. Mainstream medicine apparently overlooks the importance of particular nutrients in the causation of disease. This is a serious case of *MSA* (missing stuffs and arrows; see Chapter 1), magnified up to the level of entire areas of medicine.

Chapters 7, 8 and 10 contain case studies confirming all this. The omega-3 deficiencies are implicated not only in somatic diseases, but also in psychiatric disorders (Chapters 7 and 10). Treatment with omega-3 PUFAs is potentially beneficial in these diseases and disorders. We illustrate this here with an example of a spectacular cure.

Richardson *et al.* (1999) report the successful treatment with the food supplement eicosapentaenoic acid (EPA, an omega-3 PUFA) of a schizophrenic patient. The patient, a 30-year-old male, was exceptional since he had consistently refused to take medications. Most schizophrenic patients get strong medications with unpleasant or even dangerous side effects, to suppress debilitating symptoms. Research dealing with such patients is always problematic, because you cannot be sure whether your findings represent aspects of the disorder itself, or artefacts due to medication.

For two years prior to the study, the patient had been plagued by nasty symptoms without indications that he might recover. The study has a simple pattern. The patient was treated with EPA instead of medication. He was much improved after two months, and after six months few symptoms remained.

The example is important in several ways. First, it indicates that existing deficiencies in our diet may have grave consequences for our health, and that treatments redressing the deficiencies may have spectacular effects.

Second, the example may cast a new light on mental illnesses. These illnesses have been attributed to many sorts of causes, from genes and viruses up to bad parenting. To the extent that the illnesses follow on food deficiencies, persistent disputes about such causes would become irrelevant. It is conceivable, for example, that genes play important roles in mental illness only if our diet is inadequate.

Third, the example is a telling antidote against the view that single case studies (studies done with a single patient) cannot have much evidential force. Researchers do not hold such studies in high esteem. After all, a patient may get well after a treatment that is entirely ineffective, since recovery may reflect a natural course of the disease. We therefore have to study treatments in so-called randomised controlled trials (RCTs), in which patients receiving a treatment are compared with patients receiving a pseudo-treatment (a placebo treatment) (for details, see Chapters 4, 6 and 9). We would argue that single case studies may actually have much evidential force in some situations (see Chapter 10.6).

The present case study did not come out of the blue. Richardson *et al.* present a known theory concerning membrane biochemistry which justifies the expectation that EPA may work (details follow in Chapter 7). Furthermore, a large literature indicates that spontaneous remission of schizophrenia as described in the article should be rare. This strengthens the assumption that EPA did effect the cure. We also know that other treatments of schizophrenia are seldom as effective, and that EPA has proven beneficial effects in several other diseases associated with omega-3 deficiencies.

These indirect sources of evidence are cumulatively so strong, that the single case study compares favourably with the average RCT. Studies such as this one should stimulate research on omega-3 fatty acids in health and disease.

3.3. Poverty: The Case of Tuberculosis

Health and disease are affected by many environmental factors. The previous section illustrated effects of one factor in the biological environment, food. The present section and the next one deal with other environmental factors and interactions among them, pathogens interacting with social factors, and air pollution interacting with social factors, respectively.

We summarise in this section a case study of tuberculosis from a book by Farmer (1997) about AIDS and tuberculosis in Haiti. Farmer comes with the message that doctors need to think hard about poverty and inequality, which have a profound influence on health and disease. Many twentieth century studies show that the poor, quite simply, are sicker than the nonpoor and that this is true in both rich and poor countries (for sources, see also Patrick, 2000; Bashir, 2002; Nzerue *et al.*, 2002). Tuberculosis is one of Farmer's examples. In a recent, common view, it is a so-called emerging infectious disease, or rather a re-emerging disease. Tuberculosis is a serious problem since new strains of the bacterium causing it are resistant to almost all antibiotics (see also Shears, 2001; Dye and Espinal, 2001, who are not very pessimistic; Normark and Normark, 2002; for more recent research by Farmer and colleagues on drug resistance related to poverty, see Farmer, 2001; Rylko-Bauer and Farmer, 2002; Mitnick *et al.*, 2003).

The emerging infectious diseases are now catching medicine's attention after having been neglected for a long time, in the West that is. Popular optimism had it that we have almost eradicated the serious infectious diseases, barring developing countries, which could in principle follow suit. That optimism is no more. The diseases are making a threatening comeback.

Farmer notes that terminologies and data concerning the subject are often misleading. Official figures from the United States indicated that, in 1985, the trend of declining tuberculosis began to change. The decline fell to only 0.2 per cent in that year, and 1986 saw a 2.6 per cent increase in reported cases. In 1987, the decline was 1.1 per cent. Farmer's comments reveal how figures and their official interpretation can mislead us:

> This failure to improve was described by the term "excess cases," but the true dimensions of the problem, concealed in national statistics, are revealed by breaking down the "excess cases" according to other variables.
>
> For the CDC [Centers for Disease Control and Prevention], the salient variables are race, age, and geography. Basing an analysis on these variables reveals a much more disturbing pattern. During the years 1985-1987, we find no mere "failure to decline," but rather a sharp increase in tuberculosis rates among certain people in certain places. For example, nationwide the case rate increased 6.8 percent among blacks and 12.7 percent among Hispanics, although it *decreased* 4.8 percent among non-Hispanic whites. (...)
>
> It is thus clear that some groups—ethnic minorities—account for the majority of excess cases in the United States. (Farmer, 1997: 48)

These data together with other findings demonstrate that the perception of tuberculosis as a re-emerging or resurging disease is inconsiderate of realities experienced by particular minorities. In some groups and in some areas, the disease had never disappeared. Some have had to cope with it all their lives.

Data of modern epidemiology that represent disease incidence in general ways are often a dangerous form of *MSA*. We would add to Farmer's comments that details missed may be crucial not only for the minorities, but also for the population at large, which may run risks from unanticipated sources. Other books, for example the classic by Garrett (1994), emphasise this, whereas Farmer's concern is more with the underprivileged.

Considering the persistence of tuberculosis, Farmer (1997:

Chapter 9) distinguishes two common modes, each with many variants, of causal explanation offered by social scientists. On the one hand are those who associate persistence mainly with patient-related factors. On the other hand are those who target shortcomings of health care delivery. We also have perspectives from epidemiology, which focus on two causal factors: the advent of AIDS, and the emergence of tuberculosis strains showing multiple drug resistance. The drug resistance is often attributed to the failure of patients to comply with adequate drug prescriptions or to inadequacies in the prescriptions. This concurs with the views of social scientists.

Farmer's detailed analysis of the situation in Haiti demonstrates that these approaches are misleadingly one-sided. The case of Haiti reveals complicated relationships between individual agency and structural violence. Some patients cannot comply with treatment regimes owing to forces beyond their control:

> The biomedical literature displays a certain delicacy in discussing this problem. In the largest Haitian series in which drug susceptibilities were examined, we read only that "primary drug resistance in Haiti has many probable causes, including the availability of isoniazid without prescription, past inclusion of isoniazid in cough remedies and a high default rate." Nowhere do we read about the insurmountable barriers to effective medical care faced by the overwhelming majority of Haitians. Nowhere do we read about the absence, at that time, of an efficient national tuberculosis program that could ensure detection and treatment of cases. (Farmer, 1997: 241)

More detailed analyses by social scientists are also misleading (idem: 248-249). For example, some have identified health beliefs of patients and their families as a salient cause of failing treatment programs. In these beliefs, sorcery is the root of the illness. Social scientists have assumed that lack of compliance with treatments follows on such beliefs. Farmer shows that this assumption is false. The beliefs do *not* predict adherence to therapy. Instead, compliance and treatment outcome strongly depend on access to supplemental food and income.

The passage quoted hereafter captures the essentials of Farmer's findings, which invite us to put social issues at the heart of medicine:

> Strenuous insistence on the causal role of

> culture or personality in explaining treatment failure runs the risk of conflating cultural (or psychological) difference with structural violence, leading to the immodest claims of causality in the studies described. In theory, it would be necessary to ensure full and ready access for all persons before ascribing blame for the failure to complete treatment to patient-related shortcomings. And in none of the places in which this research was conducted is full and ready access ensured. On the contrary, these settings are crying out for measures to improve the quality of care, not the quality of the patients. ... *Throughout the world, those least likely to comply are those least able to comply.* (Farmer, 1997: 254-255)

It would be a mistake to regard this as a matter of medical practice that need not affect medical science. Farmer's study implies that lack of concern for social roots of human suffering generates epidemiological models that are *scientifically* inadequate.

3.4. Air Pollution for Poor People

Environmental factors studied by biology affect health and disease, but precise evidence concerning particular factors is hard to obtain. Interactions among these factors hamper assessment, and interactions with social factors complicate the situation further. The previous section illustrated interactions between social factors and pathogens. In the present section we consider an example of social factors interacting with air pollution.

Phillimore *et al.* (2000) have analysed air pollution in Northeast England. They show that common approaches result in distorted pictures of problems with pollution. We briefly summarise their views and their conclusions.

In a common view, from science itself and from science filtered by public institutions, air pollution affects us all, irrespective of social status. This view is false. Air pollution interacts with social status in intricate ways. The situation in Teesside, a region in Northeast England, illustrates this (see also McMichael, 2000, who makes the same point in a case study of urbanisation in developing countries). Residents of towns in Teesside have a long history of exposure to air pollution from chemical industries. Phillimore *et al.* (2000) provide evidence that pollution risks reinforce rather than cut across class inequalities:

> In the past, exposure to pollution has been as unequally distributed as wealth, and affluent areas have been far less affected than poor ones. This remains true today. Moreover, there is now credible recent evidence for an effect on mortality from this exposure in poor neighbourhoods, intensifying the inequalities in health associated with other more widely acknowledged effects of poverty. (Phillimore *et al.*, 2000: 229)

The authors present three observations of how the health problems have been handled in official accounts.

First, industries and the local government have been at pains to keep control over the pollution "story." They have made many efforts to have representatives among the investigators. To the extent that impartial views from science could be delivered at all, they persistently crafted alternative accounts in keeping with vested interests.

Second, the official rival interpretations chose to disregard the connections between pollution and poverty. They one-sidedly emphasised lifestyles associated with poverty as contributory causes of cancer and respiratory diseases, and by a sleight of hand played down the possibility that pollution should be considered a possible cause.

Third, epidemiology is a difficult discipline that yields few certainties in the search for causes of disease. This raises the spectre of burden of proof. Epidemiologists tend to be cautious, but those in power often put pressure onto them to deliver strong pronouncements. Failing these, officials tend to put the burden of proof on the shoulders of the epidemiologists, while preserving potentially dangerous situations on the ground that no risks have been uncovered. It is difficult to resolve the burden of proof issue. But it is easy to see that, in disputes about it, officials have often done away with evidence to their disliking. Theirs should then be the burden of guilt.

The third point adds a new element to the view of Farmer described in the previous section. His study of tuberculosis shows that social factors should be an essential part of medicine, and the study of air pollution by Phillimore *et al.* confirms this. In addition to this, the latter study shows that we also need to study effects of social forces that adapt research to the interests of those in power.

3.5. Conclusions

1. The influence of environmental factors on health and disease is easily underrated. Environmental studies in medicine should cover biological, social and political factors.

2. Deficiencies of omega-3 polyunsaturated fatty acids (PUFAs) in modern diets contribute to many diseases. The deficiencies are often disregarded in medicine, whereas they have been described over decades in other disciplines. Evolutionary theory helps to explain the deficiencies.

3. If we disregard effects of social and political factors on health and disease, we create inadequacies not only in medical practice but also in medical theory. Social and political factors are also important in a different way: Persons with vested interests may influence research with the purpose of arriving at theories that suit them best.

4. Single case studies of patients may have much evidential force.

Chapter 4

Drugs, Psychotherapies, and Placebos

4.1. Introduction

If you catch the flu, you are able to identify the cause. A virus has seen fit to invade your body, and it has managed to multiply there. It is as simple as that. A wise initial move would then be to forego medical treatment and let the flu run its course. Flus have a tendency to disappear by themselves, and treatments may have side effects that delay recovery instead of speeding it up. However, the virus infection may also result in some secondary infection with bacteria that calls for medical treatment. That is again a simple matter. Bacteria can be killed by a great variety antibiotics, and if you are lucky, one of them will help you get rid of the secondary infection.

The description we gave is somewhat simplistic, but it captures essentials of disease in many situations. Some situations require more complicated descriptions. Here is an example. If your sister happens to suffer from a disease that causes impaired immunity, you may wish to have efforts in place to prevent that she also gets the flu. For her, the flu might become dangerous because weakened immunity and the pathogens—viruses and bacteria—could add up as causes to make her seriously ill. In your own case, the state of the immune system would also be a causal factor affecting the course of the illness, but you would have no reason to bother about it.

Considering your sister, you may wish to know how the pathogens are transmitted. Sneezes of yours may help them reach your sister by air, but they may also find their way to her via infested door knobs. All sorts of factors in the causal chain of transmission that would not usually get your attention may now become important.

As you may extend causal images of aetiology, so also can you develop more elaborate images of treatments and the effects they cause. If your sister caught the flu in spite of precautions, then considerations concerning treatments and their effects would have to be more elaborate then they were in your own case.

In medical theory and in medical practice, context-dependent selective attention to particular causal factors is normal, indeed required, because exhaustive surveys of all the causes that influence a phenomenon are impossible (see also Chapter 2.2). The example of your flu is comparatively simple, since attending to a few causal factors sufficed to understand the disease and decide about treatment. The case of your sister is more intricate. It even has us think about the role of doorknobs in the causation of disease. In some situations, we obviously have to move beyond the normal boundaries of medicine for an adequate understanding of disease. Examples in previous chapters illustrate this, as they put medicine in broader contexts. We saw, for example, that social factors such as structural violence (Chapter 3.3) and poverty (Chapter 3.4) may be significant causes of disease, to be accounted for in treatments. This is also true for psychological factors. The study of these factors should belong to the core of medicine. It would be wrong to compartmentalise patients, in theory or in practice, and to treat them as if their bodies have nothing to do with their psychology (see also Chapter 2.3).

As the previous chapters put medicine in broad contexts, our discussion of medical treatments remained succinct. The present chapter presents a more detailed account of scientific methods for assessing treatments. Most of our examples are about drugs *versus* psychotherapy in mental illnesses. They combine to show that many pitfalls lie in wait for us in the assessment of treatments. In the last section of this chapter we present a case study of cancer that illustrates important aspects of treatment, including those introduced in the previous chapters.

4.2. Randomised Controlled Trials, Drugs, and Placebos

Suppose that we wish to test a newly developed drug for the treatment of a particular disease. If we observe positive outcomes upon treating patients with the drug, we are by no means entitled to conclude that the drug works well. Instead, the observations may merely indicate, for example, that a self-limiting disease ran its natural course.

How, then, can we obtain reliable knowledge of the drug's effects? On the face of it, the answer is simple: Instead of merely studying effects of the drug in patients with the disease, we must compare patients receiving the drug with untreated patients as controls. But significant differences between treated and untreated patients would be compelling evidence only if the two groups differed with respect to the treatment and nothing else. Barring special precautions, that would not be so. If you received the treatment, your knowing it could affect the course of your disease. The behaviour of the doctor consulted by you may also influence it. Such factors may have substantial effects.

Considering this, researchers have developed a sophisticated set-up for research on medical treatments, especially drug treatments. In randomised controlled trials (RCTs), a so-called double-blind design has to ensure that our information about treatment effects is reliable. Both the doctors and the patients are blind under this design in that they do not know which patients are receiving the drug. Untreated patients receive a pseudo-treatment with a so-called placebo, a substance without pharmacological effects on the disease.

RCTs are at the centre of Evidence-Based Medicine (EBM), which aims at a rock bottom of hard science for medical research. Advocates of EBM recognise a hierarchy of evidence in which evidence from RCTs (and from systematic reviews and meta-analyses of experimental research findings) is considered hardest: This evidence is therefore at the top of the hierarchy (for further comments on EBM, see Chapters 6 and 9). But hard evidence is hard to obtain. Even RCTs with a double-blind design need not be reliable. Drugs have side effects, and if a placebo does not have side effects like those of the drug being tested, patients receiving the drug may rightly infer that they are receiving it, since they experience the side effects. Experiments have shown that this factor does affect outcomes (see for example Shapiro and Shapiro, 1997a). So we need to use "active" placebos that mimic drug side effects, but it is often difficult to realise RCTs with such placebos.

Placebo effects have been regarded as mere psychological influences (for example by Spiro, 1998). That is an odd assumption, because the idea that psychological effects could exist without a biological counterpart is at variance with modern science. Nonetheless, controversies over the issue persist (see for example the discussion in *Advances of mind-body medicine* summarised by Dienstfrey, 2000, and the discussion following the article by Moerman and Jonas, 2000, in the same issue). Many studies have shown that placebo's do affect the physiology of patients (Kirsch, 1997; Eskandari and Sternberg, 2002; Price and Soerensen, 2002). Baxter *et al.* (1992) have shown, for example, that successful psychotherapeutic treatment and successful drug treatment of obsessive-compulsive symptoms cause similar brain imagery changes.

We know that many different mechanisms contribute to placebo effects, for example conditioning by previous treatments, or responses set in motion by expected outcomes (Brody and Brody, 1997; Harrington, 1997; Bootzin and Caspi, 2002; Harrington, 2002; Kleinman *et al.*, 2002; Moerman, 2002; Siegel, 2002). But we generally do not know what factors are effective in particular cases. If we would know about this, we could use placebo treatments as genuine treatments. Shapiro and Shapiro

(1997b: 29) rightly state: “If everything were known about the aetiology of the placebo effect, the terms *placebo* and *placebo effect* would disappear and be replaced by a hugely powerful megapsychotherapy.”

The boundary between drugs and placebos is also hazy because psychological and other situational variables contribute to “biological” effects of drugs (Fisher and Greenberg, 1997; Morris 1997). For example, clinical settings and experimental settings may differ in placebo effects, the nature of the relationship between doctor and patient may have a marked effect, personality variables play a role, and the outward appearance of the medication makes a difference.

A troubling point is here that the RCT design may conceal the real power of placebos (Roberts, 1994 and 1995). Patients in an RCT, knowing that they may not receive the real drug, may have comparatively low expectations that obstruct the healing process, whereas high expectations in a clinical setting have a positive effect. Roberts mentions treatments with high success scores in clinical settings that later turned out to be entirely ineffective.

RCT outcomes may also mislead us as they need not allow extrapolation to the population we wish to consider. Extrapolations are legitimate only if the samples studied are representative for the population. They may not be legitimate, for example, as a result of comorbidity (for reference, see Greenberg, 1997: 60-61). Comorbidity means that, in addition to the disease being studied, patients have another disease also. High levels of comorbidity are common. In some psychiatric disorders the level may be around 50 per cent. It is misleading to regard this as a fact of nature, because shortcomings in classifications of disorders may generate artificial comorbidities (Carson, 1997; see also Chapter 2). Considering comorbidity, we face a difficult choice concerning patient inclusion in RCTs. If we include patients who exhibit comorbidity, we get a heterogeneous sample of patients and of treatment effects. But if we exclude them, we may get a comparatively healthy group of subjects with unrepresentative, beneficial treatment effects. Thus, we would overestimate the effects.

All in all, RCTs would generate fully reliable conclusions only if they complied with a host of sophisticated methodological criteria that can hardly be jointly satisfied. This does not imply that we should do away with RCTs, though. Pincus (2002) presents an extensive overview of limitations of RCTs, but he keeps endorsing them as a valuable tool of research. We concur with his view since *all* sources of evidence have limitations. The best strategy would be to supplement RCT outcomes with evidence from sources that have different strengths and weaknesses. For example, single case studies may yield valuable evidence, especially if observed treatment effects fit with scientific theories (see the single case study of schizophrenia described in Chapter 3.5). Theories added to data are a valid source of evidence.

In some situations, RCTs have been invaluable. Cases are known, for example, in which alleged positive effects of a drug "disappeared" as methodological sophistication of controlled trials increased. That should count as *prima facie* evidence against the drug. RCTs with a high methodological quality may also count against views based on clinical judgment and common sense. But it would be foolish to dispense with clinical judgment and common sense altogether.

4.3. Problems with Drugs

So far we only considered problems with placebos in a theoretical way (we continue theoretical considerations in Chapter 9). Let us have a look at how the problems work out in practice.

Greenberg and Fisher (1997) provide an excellent survey of antidepressants such as lithium and selective serotonin re-uptake inhibitors (SSRIs). Many RCTs have resulted in positive effects of antidepressant medications. However, most studies are unreliable, because they were done with inert placebos rather than active placebos with side effects (see the previous section). Studies with active placebos typically revealed minor effects only or no effects at all. This alone suggests that many common drug treatments of depression are problematic (for additional comments and references, see Chapters 6.3 and 10.2).

For several reasons, evidence from RCTs with active placebos need not be conclusive either. First, patients with particular features may have to be excluded, so that the RCTs are not representative. Second, putative beneficial effects may be due to side effects of the drugs. For example, if the drugs cause you to have headaches, this may help you forget about problems that were causing your depression. Third, outcome measures cause problems. Symptoms of depression and other psychiatric disorders cannot be measured in a simple way. Physical quantities such as, say, body length, can be measured in a direct way. But the manifold mental symptoms studied by psychiatrists can only be assessed with qualitative or semiquantitative measures. Researchers commonly use a so-called score, which combines values attributed to all sorts of symptoms. Thus we get a kind of "rating" based on decisions about the relevance of different symptoms. This is a potential source of arbitrariness and bias (for details, see Greenberg and Fisher, 1997). Beneficial effects of antidepressants observed in RCTs are often based on clinician ratings.

Effects assessed by patients rating their own outcomes have been less beneficial. The patient-rated measures turned out to be methodologically superior in comparison with the clinician-rated measures. This is an additional reason for being sceptical about antidepressants.

If RCTs compellingly showed that an antidepressant would be superior to a placebo, this would by no means imply that it should be a treatment of choice. A different treatment could well outperform the antidepressant. Indeed, comparative studies of drugs *versus* psychotherapy in depression have demonstrated that psychotherapy is often at least as effective as medication. Psychotherapy is not the only alternative to common medications. Particular essential fatty acids that are lacking in most diets in our culture, have beneficial effects in depression and other mental illnesses (for details, see Chapters 7 and 10).

Recent research confirms all the points made by Greenberg and Fisher (1997). Kirsch *et al.* (2002) argue in a comprehensive target article that the effects of antidepressants appear to be minor at best. Responses by commentators following the article are not unanimous, but overall they indicate that evidence of substantial effects is still lacking. Furthermore, negative side effects have been reported in many studies. It is amazing that the consumption of antidepressants keeps increasing against hundreds of negative reports. The discrepancy is explained in part by the common confusion in research of statistical significance with clinical relevance. Small differences between treatment outcomes and placebo outcomes may be statistically significant while being clinically irrelevant. Bias in favour of the drugs is increased further by selective reporting. Most studies are funded by the pharmaceutical industry. Negative studies normally remain unpublished, and the industry is often allowed to market products on the basis of a few positive studies, even if many other studies have failed to demonstrate effects. The role of the industry is considered in greater detail in Chapters 6.3 and 8.

Neuroleptics, also called antipsychotics, are another major category of drugs used in psychiatry. They invite even more negative comments (for a survey, see Cohen, 1997, and Healy, 2002, whose book is reviewed in Chapter 6.3). The drugs are used against psychoses, especially in schizophrenia. They may induce a general deterioration of mental functioning characterised, for example, by apathy. The so-called antipsychotic effect is then at best a sign of this deterioration. Some studies have shown that neuroleptics decrease relapse rates if patients keep being treated with them after being dismissed from a hospital or psychiatric ward. However, this seemingly beneficial effect was observed only in comparison with patients subject to relatively sudden withdrawal from the drugs. A more gradual withdrawal reduces the chances of relapse. In addition to the adverse psychological effects, the neuroleptics also have serious neurological side effects. Considering older neuroleptics, psychiatrists recognise this. They have suggested that newer neuroleptics, the so-called atypical antipsychotics, are less problematic, but available evidence does not support this (see for example Geddes *et al.*, 2000; Burns, 2001; Glassman, 2002; Llorca *et al.*, 2002; Meltzer *et al.*, 2002). Much research on neuroleptics has a poor quality. High quality studies indicate that the effectiveness of the neuroleptics is vastly overrated. Psychotherapy combined with help by laypersons may often be a better option. Medications used in anxiety disorders invite similar comments (see the review by Danton and Antonuccio, 1997).

Overall, a critical analysis of the literature proves that irresponsible prescriptions of psychotropic medications are common (for additional data, comments and references, see Jacobs, 1995 and 1999). Drugs may at times be a good choice in some severe disorders. By and large, however, drug therapy should be an option of the last resort. This does not imply, though, that benefits of psychotherapy should be accepted as a matter of course. The survey in the next section shows that psychotherapy has problems of its own.

4.4. Conundrums of Psychotherapy

Psychotherapies come in many kinds, hundreds of them in fact. The assessment of the therapies is mostly done in a discipline called psychotherapy research. The overall results of assessments are amazing. Most therapies have modest beneficial effects, but the factors regarded as effective by adherents of a particular therapeutic mode are seldom operative. Instead, factors shared by therapies, for example a caring attitude of the therapist, appear to bring about the beneficial effect. In a way, therefore, psychotherapies are placebo treatments writ large. Dawes (1994) shows in an extensive review that the therapies, if effective at all, work by way of "non-specific" factors (see also Russell, 1994, and the volume edited by Soldz and McCullough, 2000, which addresses tensions between research and practice).

More disturbing facts are also revealed by Dawes. The experience and the formal credentials of therapists are unrelated to success rates, and lay therapists, after a brief training, often perform as well as professional therapists. How can we explain this odd finding? Dawes argues that essential prerequisites for improvement by learning are mostly absent in work done by therapists. In therapies, they cannot easily identify and understand mistakes, and they lack a clear mechanism to correct mistakes.

Research has also shown that diagnoses and predictions of therapy outcomes by therapists relying on clinical judgment are poor in comparison with diagnoses and predictions done with statistical methods. This is explained by biases that are common in intuitive human judgments. If we need to assess a complicated phenomenon because it calls for actions on our part, we base our judgments on heuristics that suit practical purposes. For example, with the so-called availability heuristic we search our memory for instances similar to the one at hand, and with the so-called representativeness heuristic we look for a stereotype for the case at hand. Heuristics are profitable rules of thumb, but they have limitations. However useful in daily life, they may lead us astray in many situations. Psychotherapy research indicates that judgements based on heuristics need not work well in psychotherapies.

The results of psychotherapy research, however telling, do not imply that intuitive clinical judgements are always inferior to formal decision procedures. Nor do they imply that common sense should give way to science whenever that is possible. Intuition and common sense informed by experience work well, for example, in the recognition of bird species by field biologists. The comparative values of intuition, common sense and formal reasoning are context-dependent (Kleinmuntz, 1990). Considering the treatment of mental illnesses, we hold intuition and common sense in high esteem. It is true that they do not work well in professionalised psychotherapeutics. But this does not imply that they are the root cause of poor professionalisation. We conjecture that it is often the other way round, as overshoots of professionalisation may dull intuition and common sense.

4.5. Putting it All Together: The Case of Cancer

The assessment of medical treatments is complicated, nightmarishly so at times. That much is obvious by now. Medicine uses many quantitative methods to assess treatments. Prospective epidemiological studies yield valuable evidence, for example. We have only considered RCTs, because they are commonly regarded as the best source of evidence. But it turns out that even RCTs have many theoretical and practical limitations. RCTs and Evidence-Based Medicine in general are nonetheless indispensable in medicine. How indeed could medicine be a rational undertaking if we did not aim at an evidential basis backed by science? Goodman (2003) has eloquently made this point in an analysis of strengths and weaknesses of Evidence-Based Medicine. He argues that evidence should not be defined in an overly narrow way. We would indeed suggest that evidence from RCTs and other quantitative approaches has to be supplemented with evidence from other sources inclusive of common sense.

Our first priority would be with the search for *MSA* (missing stuffs and arrows, see Chapter 1). Research on treatments, however sophisticated, may miss the mark when a significant factor, or indeed a significant discipline, is disregarded. We do not mean that research should always account for all the factors that may affect a problem under investigation. That is impossible, increasingly so as scientific knowledge accumulates with an ever increasing pace (a problem discussed extensively in Chapter 5). The issue is rather that ideas existing in some domain may have a significant bearing on subjects in another domain where the ideas are disregarded. Examples in this book indicate that this is a common phenomenon (see especially Chapters 3, 5 and 7). On top of this, existing power structures in our society may suppress potentially valuable research of medical treatments (for examples, see Chapters 3, 6, 8 and 10).

The case study of cancer that follows illustrates these sources of bias. To start with, we comment on an impressive recent book by Williams (2002), who survived a brain tumour of a nasty variety that usually causes death within a few months after the first symptoms appear. After surgery, rests of Williams' tumour started to grow again. Williams decided to do an extensive search of the literature, and he consulted many professionals about possible therapies. In stages, he developed a therapy of his own based on a great variety of sources. In brief, he combined many different treatments including chemotherapies, and also promising treatments from complementary and alternative medicine (CAM). Meanwhile, he had to fight the medical establishment as his ideas were at variance with standard therapies.

Williams presents a valuable analysis of Evidence-Based Medicine in the United States. Considering clinical trials, he criticises the set-up that is commonly accepted in cancer research. For a new treatment to be marketed, it must be approved by the Food and Drug Administration (FDA). Approval is contingent on a successful completion of three phases. In phase-I trials, the safety profile of the new drug is investigated by experimenting with dosages. Phase-II trials are small-scale tests of treatment efficacy, often done in a single treatment centre. As phase-II outcomes may not be representative for the target population, large-scale phase-III trials are subsequently done at many centres. Williams notes many problems with this set-up and with its implementation. We have already mentioned two of them. The large scale of the phase-III trials results in much heterogeneity among patients (see Section 2), and statistically significant treatment effects need not be clinically relevant (see Section 3). Williams also notes that many promising treatments do not reach the stage of phase-III trials, which are expensive, as the industry would not make money out of them. For example, promising food supplements are not patentable. The medical community also tends to stay with "proven" treatments, which in many cases prolong life a little bit at the cost of nasty side effects.

Williams backs up his own approach with theoretical considerations that appear to be eminently rational. As to chemotherapy, for example, he has focussed on drugs with a comparatively low toxicity. That allowed him to combine more of them than most practitioners would have it. Also, he took drugs with different mechanisms of action. Sensibly, he reasoned that this would enhance the chances that the tumour responded. He considered that the distinction of "proven" and "unproven" therapies is an outdated, rigid dichotomy, a thesis which we endorse. The dichotomy is based on one-sided choice of sources of evidence, and it does not account for discrepancies between statistical significance and clinical relevance. In making choices from therapies, Williams did his own appraisal of the evidence.

A strong point of Williams' book is that it offers a well-reasoned alternative for existing research into treatments. Williams argues that treatments should be individualised. That is best done by taking patient characteristics into account. Statistical averages from large-scale trials are meaningless if we do not account for heterogeneity among patients. Hence we should use a databases that allow us to have patients in subgroups with similar characteristics. If this is done in an accurate way, we may even dispense with phase-III trials. In the view of the cancer establishment, this is a revolutionary proposal.

Williams' view does not amount to a crusade against Evidence-Based Medicine as such. He rather argues that existing methods of searching for evidence are flawed. We would distinguish here between Evidence-Based Medicine as a dominant, canonised entity, and evidence-based medicine, the variety of medicine that aims at evidence in support of medical science and medical practice. The acceptance of evidence-based medicine by no means entails the acceptance of Evidence-Based Medicine.

Williams did not consider psychotherapy. We supplement his views with an application to cancer of the main theme of this chapter, drugs *versus* psychotherapy. The assessment of either kind of therapy is complicated. To fully understand the therapies, we need to know much more than we do now about the interaction of our biology and our psychology. This interaction is studied in many interdisciplines, most notably psychoimmunology, also called, more accurately, psychoneuroimmunology, or even psychoneuroendocrinoimmunology, here abbreviated as PNEI (for references, see Leonard and Miller, 1995; Martin, 1997; Rabin, 1999; Goodkin and Visser, 2000; Koenig and Cohen, 2002; Sivik *et al.*, 2002).

At the centre of PNEI is the interaction of mental and somatic processes, especially the influence of stress on the immune system. Terms such as "immune system" should actually be regarded as misnomers to be used for convenience of terminology. Our bodies do not really have an immune system, a nervous system and an endocrine system. These systems are actually a single system. The three "systems" are interconnected by numerous substances, pathways and processes, and they are influenced by many psychological factors and environmental factors. This implies that highly general claims about effects of drugs and psychotherapies are impossible. RCTs have value, but their outcomes are valid only under conditions that were realised during the trials. We should expect that outcomes of different studies will often conflict. Hence, evidence from RCTs has to be supplemented with evidence from qualitative research and commonsensical considerations (for details, see Chapter 9).

An old issue in PNEI is whether psychosocial factors may affect the immune system so as to increase the life span of cancer patients. The book edited by Lewis *et al.* (2002) presents an excellent survey of the issue. The analyses in the book cast doubts on old claims that cancer can be influenced via mental processes, for example in psychotherapy. Much research about this was methodologically flawed. Some recent investigations yielded positive results, but conflicting findings are common. All in all, the jury is still out. We would apply Williams' line of reasoning to the issue of PNEI and cancer. Cancer treatments have to be individualised, and research into treatments has to account for heterogeneity among patients. Studies with the ordinary RCT format can but generate conflicting results, because patient samples will be different in different studies. Cunningham (2002) has indeed argued that RCTs in research on psychosocial aspects of cancer are best replaced by qualitative correlational studies that take features of individual patients into account.

Entirely different approaches of cancer treatments exist in CAM, complementary and alternative medicine (some of which are reviewed by Williams). We find here much quackery, highly promising treatments, and everything in between. Moss has been one the most important champions of sound research on CAM therapies. In 1977, he was fired by the famous Memorial Sloan-Kettering Cancer Center for opposing their cover-up of positive data on the drug laetrile. After that, he has long been active in attempts to get sound research on CAM therapies off the ground. In his book (1996, updated edition) he reveals how official governmental organisations and industries opposed this research. Clinics that provided evidence of favourable outcomes with alternative therapies have been ransacked or closed down, the evidence has been disregarded in official reports, data have been falsified, funds have been allocated mainly to research programs serving persons and organisations with vested interests, research mandated by Congress has not been carried out, and so forth.

These things are seldom considered in official publications about cancer presented as objective, value-neutral science. They may shed a new light on all the research about psychosocially supportive therapies. Research on these therapies, if conducted in accordance with strict RCT standards, is almost always carried out with patients who also get treatments along "orthodox" lines, for example chemotherapy. Results obtained in this way are valid only for situations in which orthodox treatments are provided as well. What would happen if we combined psychosocial treatments with promising CAM therapies? Nobody knows, since methodologically adequate research on the matter has been scarce. To a large extent, this situation has been created and sustained by persons and organisations with power to determine research strategies and the allocation of funds.

In addition to psychotherapies and CAM therapies, we should also consider diet therapies as a supplementary treatment of cancer. There can be no doubt that our current diets are unnatural and that they foster many diseases, cancers among them (see Chapter 7). Shortages of particular fatty acids, especially omega-3 acids, are an important culprit. At the very least, changes in our diet can help us prevent cancer. But the signs are also that these fatty acids represent a valuable supplemental treatment modality (for references, see Chapter 7.4).

We end this survey with one example from the book by Moss (his Chapter 7) of a promising alternative therapy that faded to the background as it did not fit in with received opinions of the cancer establishment. In the late nineteenth century, a young New York City surgeon, William Coley, stumbled across an intriguing phenomenon. He discovered a patient with an advanced case of cancer who, apparently on his deathbed, was infected with the bacterium *Streptococcus pyogenes* causing erysipelas, a severe and sometimes life-threatening infection of the skin. The patient recovered and, to the amazement of the doctors, left his deathbed, his tumour having shrunk.

Coley subsequently treated cancer patients by inoculating them with the bacterium, and he obtained impressive cure rates with several cancers. The bacterium apparently produces a toxin that can act as a potent drug against cancer. It boosts the immune system by association with the so-called tumour necrosis factor (TNF). A neat RCT conducted in 1982 by Nauts confirmed the Coley approach. After that the approach fell into oblivion. Here is how Moss ends his chapter: "The fact is, a century after Coley's initial success it remains nearly impossible for a patient to opt for this extraordinary therapy in any form." After the appearance of the book by Moss, the situation has changed somewhat. The value of Coley's work has ultimately been rediscovered. Hoption Cann *et al.* (2002) suggest that Coley's approach may still represent one of the most effective immunotherapies for cancer, and some research is being done to refine the approach (see, for example, Hobohm, 2001).

Some would argue that the situation has improved after the appearance of Moss' book, but recent studies of cancer research (Epstein, 1998; Hess, 1999) and studies in other areas of medicine (see Chapters 7, 8 and 10) suggest that, overall, vested interests keep determining the course of much medical research. Let us hope for more democratic politics to decrease bias against the interests of patients.

4.6. Conclusions

1. Modern drug treatments are allegedly based on sound science, realised in randomised controlled trials (RCTs). But such trials face thorny methodological problems which are underrated in psychiatry.

2. Overmedication is common in psychiatry. Methodologically sophisticated research indicates that the use of drugs in psychiatry is often problematic and that psychotherapy is often a better option.

3. Psychotherapies may represent an effective treatment of mental illnesses, but their effects may not ensue from specific factors deemed effective by therapists. A humane approach of patients may be one of the most important factors.

4. Methodological research indicates that the formal expertise of psychotherapists does not correlate well with treatment results. This suggests that it may be wise to cherish common sense in psychotherapy. But research has also revealed weaknesses of common sense in clinical judgments. We have to strike a balance and use miscellaneous sources of knowledge.

5. Problems with the assessment of drug treatments are aggravated by bias in research serving the interests of industries rather than patients. This problem is exemplified by cancer research. It is to be hoped that the balance of interests can be redressed by democratic means.

6. Promising cancer therapies have been disregarded by the medical establishment. Research on therapies is one-sided owing to inadequate procedures of approving therapies for the market. Research on the merits of therapies from complementary and alternative medicine (CAM) should be stimulated.

Chapter 5

Migraine: A Plethora of Disorders

5.1. Introduction

Migraine is a common disease which is often misunderstood. That is, persons who suffer from it are often misunderstood, since many people would not regard it as a genuine disorder. Cady (1999) reports that an estimated 23 million Americans suffer from disabling migraines. But only a minority are diagnosed. Underrecognition, underconsultation and undertreatment are common (see also Sheftell and Tepper, 2002).

Considering what medical science has to say about migraine, we can add theoretical nonunderstanding to personal misunderstanding. The scientific literature about migraine is large, and recent research has unveiled numerous mechanisms at the cellular and the molecular level which are operative in some, never in all migraine phenomena. No integrative view exists, or, more accurately, many integrative theories have been proposed without being united.

We do not think that an integrative theory is feasible, since migraine is a heterogeneous collection of phenomena. But we do aim to present a fresh outlook. The materials presented here show that many potential contributions from biology have fallen by the wayside, and we would like to see them on the way again. Taken as a whole, the staggering quantity of scientific details concerning migraine could suggest that potentially promising areas of research on migraine should be covered, but that is not so. As detailed knowledge accumulates in the life sciences, blank areas accumulate as well. Existing research is rich, prolific and unbalanced. Considering migraine, we try to contribute to a restoration of balance by locating miscellaneous gaps in ongoing research.

We follow the lead of Swanson, a specialist of scientific documentation in medicine. Over many years, he has developed methods of locating missing links in the literature, with so much success that he received an award for his work (Swanson, 2001). His primary tool is automated search by way of key words to find unconnected literatures dealing with similar phenomena (Swanson, 1990; Swanson and Smalheiser, 1997 and 1999). This often leads to the formulation of new, fruitful hypotheses. Two of his case studies happen to fit with the subject of the present chapter.

In one study, Swanson identified articles showing that dietary fish oils lead to certain blood and vascular changes, and also articles with evidence that similar changes might benefit patients with Raynaud's phenomenon (reduced blood flow in small arteries of the hands, which easily become cold as a result) (Swanson, 1986 and 1987). The two sets of articles had never been connected. Taken jointly, they generate the hypothesis that dietary fish oil may benefit Raynaud patients. This was indeed confirmed in subsequent research.

A later case study undertaken by Swanson concerns migraine (Swanson, 1988 and 1991). An extensive search of unconnected literatures resulted in the hypothesis that magnesium deficiency is presumably an important causal factor in migraine headache. This made us curious, and we have done a brief search of more recent literature concerning magnesium and migraine. We report here some results as an aside showing that Swanson's approach may help set us on new, fruitful tracks. Johnson (2001) reports that the importance of magnesium is easily overlooked as it is by far the least abundant electrolyte in blood plasma. Yet, it subserves many body functions. Magnesium deficiency is common, and it may cause a great variety of disorders. Recent research does confirm that magnesium may be important in migraine (see for example Boska *et al.*, 2002; Mauskop *et al.*, 2002).

Unfortunately, Johnson argues, the mere use of magnesium as a food supplement need not redress deficiencies, because magnesium metabolism depends on many variables. These have to be taken into account in the development of therapies. This point deserves to be generalised. In research on causal factors in the pathogenesis and the treatment of diseases, indeed in research in general, we have to keep the factors studied within manageable bounds. Thus, in experimental work we keep many factors at some constant level, while varying the factors we wish to study. This kind of rigor strengthens evidential force, but at the same time it restricts the domain in which our findings have evidential force. If factors kept constant were set at different levels, we could obtain different results. The implications of this banal truth are far-reaching, and they are vastly underrated. As sophistication of research at the molecular level increases, we have to deal with increasing numbers of factors, and this restricts the domains in which our findings are applicable. This may well be an important cause of failed connections among literatures.

To our surprise, Swanson did not forge connections between the case studies on Raynaud's phenomenon and migraine. Migraine is often associated with Raynaud's phenomenon (examples of recent sources:

Voulgari *et al.*, 2000; Constantinescu, 2002). That is not surprising as the vascular system is involved in either case. Many of the blood and vascular changes observed in Raynaud's phenomenon should also play a role in migraine. Furthermore, fish oil may be a promising treatment option not only in Raynaud's phenomenon, but also in migraine. We will come back to this.

Swanson's work was unknown to us until recently. One of us (WJS) has followed his type of method over the years, albeit in a more intuitive fashion, and with more emphasis on generalist work relying on textbooks from many disciplines. The present chapter illustrates how this works out in the case of migraine. We begin with a survey of elements from current views in biomedicine, and subsequently introduce in stages items that do not receive the attention they deserve.

5.2. Problems With Classification

A recent book by Davidoff (2002) is presumably the most comprehensive text about migraine. Davidoff suffers from migraine himself, and as a medical professional he has for a long time specialised in this disorder. Our survey of elements from recent research on migraine draws to a large extent on his book.

For research to get off the ground we have to characterise the subject to be investigated. That is already a tall order in the case of migraine, since it represents not a single disorder but a collection of disorders with diffuse boundaries. This is a common sort of situation in medicine that restricts the feasibility of general theories (see Chapter 2).

Davidoff is acutely aware of this (see Chapter 1 of his book). He decides to use whenever possible the classification published in 1988 by the Headache Classification Committee of the International Headache Society (IHS), which is generally regarded as the best system. This classification recognises seven subtypes of migrainous headaches. The vast majority of these headaches belong to two subtypes, migraine without aura and migraine with aura. Auras are neurological phenomena that may take many forms, for example abnormalities of vision. The IHS classification stipulates that several characteristic features are requisite for a diagnosis of migraine, for example a limited duration of attacks (4 to 72 hours), intense unilateral pain and nausea.

Davidoff notes that this classification, indeed any classification of headaches, is arbitrary in some respects. The criteria suit research purposes at the population level; they have been used for example in almost all drug trials. But they do not work very well in the evaluation of patients in clinical settings, since the IHS definitions "specify only typical, homogeneous headache syndromes, when in fact many transitional types of headaches have migrainous features, but may or may not be migrainous" (Davidoff, 2002: 6). The classification is also problematic in other respects. Many patients suffer from several types of migraine, so that multiple diagnoses apply to them; contrary to the classification, migraines and tension-type headaches do not in fact exist as neatly separable categories; and so forth. In brief, "migraine" is an abstract word for a heterogeneous category of phenomena.

5.3. Some Hypotheses

Many hypotheses have been proposed to explain migraine. Wolff, in a monograph published in 1963, was the first to provide a comprehensive account (see Davidoff, 2002: 190). He proposed that migraine is primarily a problem of the blood circulation. According to him, constriction of particular blood vessels in the brain and blood vessels outside the skull, set in motion a chain of events that ultimately causes the headache and phenomena associated with it. Local lack of oxygen in the brain would cause aura phenomena. An initial vasoconstriction (constriction of blood vessels) would cause sterile inflammation of vessels, followed by reactive vasodilatation (dilatation of vessels). The vasodilatation would cause stretching of nerve endings in the wall of blood vessels and thereby generate the pain.

Wolff's hypothesis has been popular over decades, but it turned out not to explain all migraine phenomena. Nowadays, the neuronal hypothesis has many more adherents. This hypothesis postulates processes in particular nerve cells in the brain that secondarily cause changes in the vascular system.

Davidoff argues that the two hypotheses are not necessarily competitors. Both the vascular system and the nervous system are anyhow involved, and research has meanwhile uncovered numerous mechanisms with a role for both systems in migraine attacks. For example, Wolff's idea concerning stretched nerve endings has taken a more specific form. In migraine, vasodilatation appears to stimulate pain receptors in blood vessel walls in a particular area of the brain, the dura. A phenomenon called cortical spreading depression, which is presumably associated with aura phenomena, is another example of complex interactions between the vascular system and the nervous system. Spreading depression has been monitored in detail in experimental animals. If the cortex of the brain is stimulated in particular ways, nerve cell activity and blood flow decrease.

The effect spreads slowly over a larger area of the cortex. The activity of the nerve cells is soon restored, but blood flow may remain off balance for as long as an hour.

The vascular system and the nervous system cannot provide the entire story of migraine. Hormones also play a crucial role. Much attention has been paid to serotonin, a neurotransmitter hormone (Davidoff, 2002: Chapter 12; see also the next section). The serotonin hypothesis of migraine allots an important role to particular blood cells, the platelets, which contain almost all the serotonin stored in the blood. In some cases at least, migraine attacks are associated with changes in platelet serotonin, which may generate pain attacks by affecting brain biochemistry.

The themes considered so far are all in Davidoff's book. We supplement them with some details from other sources which suggest that the immune system plays a role in migraine. Davidoff does not pay much attention to the immune system. The system should be important as migraine appears to involve local sterile inflammation of blood vessels in particular areas of the brain. The inner lining of the blood vessels, the endothelium, plays a major role in the inflammation (Appenzeller, 1991). Irritation of the endothelium plays a part, for example, in the triggering of aura phenomena. The irritation results in local aggregation and adhesion of blood cells, especially platelets, at the endothelium. Hanington *et al.* (1981) have indeed called migraine a platelet disorder (see also Mezei, 2000). Dreier *et al.* (2002) managed to show, for the first time, that secretion of a substance called endothelin-1 by the endothelium can induce spreading depression in rats. Thus, this substance may be one of the factors inducing auras. Other blood cells, especially T-cells of the immune system, are also affected in migraine. Martelletti *et al.* (1989) observed that, in food-induced migraine, changes occurred in immune complexes in the blood and in T-cell numbers, and Empl *et al.* (1999) observed in migraine patients changes in T-cells interacting with the endothelium.

The review by Flammer *et al.* (2001) is an eye-opener in the matter of vasoconstriction and vasodilatation. They discuss the phenomenon of sudden vasoconstriction, vasospasm. They state that all sorts of factors may cause vasoconstriction in a great variety of disorders, migraine among them. Characteristically, blood levels of endothelin-1 are high in patients experiencing vasoconstriction. The authors notice that the clinical impact of vascular dysregulation has been appreciated only in the last few years. This review implies in our view that we should not be concerned overmuch with the search for mechanisms that are specific for migraine. A variety of different diseases may share aetiological factors and general mechanisms, and the study of what is shared may yield a basis for finding details that count in individual diseases.

5.4. Drugs, Placebos, and RCTs

The popularity of the serotonin hypothesis is of a piece with the recent emergence of triptans, drugs affecting serotonin metabolism that are commonly used to treat migraine attacks (Davidoff, 2002: Chapter 16). Davidoff presents an extensive survey which also covers other drugs that are potentially useful in migraine (see also the review by Diamond and Wenzel, 2002). No drug benefits all patients on all occasions, and some drugs may have undesirable side effects. If drugs are to be used, the doctor and the patient often need to try out many of them before an apparently suitable one is found. Davidoff repeatedly argues that treatments should be individualised in view of heterogeneity among migraine patients, and that a reconstruction of the patient's history provides the most valuable clues for diagnosis and treatment. Case histories are important because all sorts of factors, many of them concerning life styles, may trigger migraine attacks. Aetiologies, just like explanatory hypotheses, and effects of treatments do not universally apply to all patients.

Davidoff (2002: 296-298) notes that research on drug treatments for migraine has uncovered clear placebo responses, at times responses with a dramatic magnitude. But no general tendency has emerged, since responses depend on many situational factors. Medical professionals commonly agree that we have to account for placebo effects in the study of treatments, preferably by randomised controlled trials (RCTs) with a double-blind set-up (see Chapter 4). RCTs are the core of so-called Evidence-Based Medicine, which is replacing the older tradition of acquiring knowledge through clinical experience. RCTs are a valuable tool, but they have disadvantages. Considering headache medications, Davidoff argues that extrapolation of data from RCTs to the clinic is difficult. RCTs need to have rigor. For example, the patient samples to be studied must be clearly defined. That is a difficult requirement in the case of migraine. As rigor increases, the chances are that the patient samples studied in RCTs will not be representative for the populations of patients treated in medical practice. Furthermore, patients recruited in clinical trials have the advantage of additional clinic visits and laboratory tests. This causes biased clinical outcomes.

Physicians, in view of such problems, will have to find out to what extent their patients resemble patients in a trial of a drug they may wish to prescribe. The RCTs themselves do not provide the clues which the physicians need. Hence, the value of quantitative information from RCTs is limited (see also Chapter 9). Davidoff also notes that further bias may be introduced by the inclination of journal editors to publish positive results more than negative results. We add to all this that the pharmaceutical industry, which has a major share in the funding of research, may be responsible for an even greater bias. We have not found evidence of this in literature on medications for migraine, but this is a distinct possibility, since the industry has enhanced the use of inappropriate medications in other cases (see Chapters 6.3, 8 and 10).

Bias concerning drug treatments may arise also as some potentially valuable treatments with food supplements would not yield profits for the industry. The role of these food supplements is considered in Section 7.

5.5. Folk Biology and Common Sense

Biomedical research of migraine has generated much detailed, technical information. This information is helpful, but it may also obscure the feasibility of useful, more elementary approaches of migraine. Considering non-pharmacological treatments, we outline here an elementary way of thinking that may benefit some migraine patients. First, we briefly discuss some aspects of physical therapy that fit with experiences of our own with migraine patients.

Migraine episodes are often initiated by trigger points in muscles, called myofascial trigger points, of the head, neck or shoulders (Davidoff, 2002: 110-111 and 307). These points are easily located as they lie in thickened muscle areas. A chronic or an acute overload of the muscles can provoke a so-called myofascial pain syndrome that may be regarded as a variety of migraine. The syndrome hardly responds to drug treatments. Patients suffering from it may benefit from physical therapy that restores muscle function. Davidoff also mentions here postural training. Maintaining a good posture is an essential element of a conscious, healthy lifestyle.

We add to Davidoff's remarks some considerations deriving from common sense and elementary biology. Migraine may be affected by patterns of blood circulation and allied physiological processes in the entire body. For example, if after waking up you begin your day with a ham and eggs breakfast, your stomach will be set to work and it will receive a rich supply of blood. As blood cannot be in different places at the same time, the supply to other organs, the brain for example, may be diminished accordingly. Furthermore, your movements will be limited during breakfast, so that metabolites in your muscles which accumulated during sleep are not easily removed. The lack of movement also tends to slow down blood circulation. These considerations suggest that some exercise before breakfast should improve your condition, so as to decrease the risk of a migraine attack. In addition to this, if you do suffer from myofascial pain points, some form of massage may be helpful.

Drink should be as important as food. Your blood circulation will be enhanced if you have a few glasses of water before breakfast, for example. You will know about getting thirsty after eating sweets or salty things. The habit of doing this sets in motion physiological processes that affect the water balance in our bodies. This may call for compensation by drinking. The water balance affects blood circulation. All in all, we would assume that experimentally altering habits of eating and drinking may provide clues for the abatement of migraine. We have not uncovered literature exploring these mundane things.

Next, we would suggest that the deliberate use of muscles in areas where blood circulation is limited may be helpful. If your feet are cold, you may consider moving them in all possible directions, by rotation, stretching, and so forth, and massaging muscles of your calves. The circulation of blood is also affected, markedly so, by regimes of temperature exposure. Repeated exposure of the skin to low temperatures enhances skin responsiveness, which decreases suffering from cold hands or cold feet. The general idea is that frequent exposure to alternating heat and cold has beneficial effects on blood circulation.

Among friends and acquaintances, one of us (WJS) has often tried out this kind of thing. Experiments mostly had positive results. For example, I (WJS) witnessed the disappearance of a bout of Raynaud-like complaints (cold hands and cold feet due to restricted blood flow) within a few minutes upon brief massage and physical exercise. Likewise in some cases for severe migraine attacks, after massage of painful muscles. In parentheses, I note that I have also witnessed alternative treatments that may be labelled as "psychic healing" and "aura healing." In some cases, patients reported instantaneous disappearance of severe headache after a very brief treatment. This suggests that possibilities may exist for effective treatments beyond existing scientific worldviews (see Chapter 12).

The anecdotes do not have much evidential force. But they may represent a potentially valuable way of thinking which appears to be rare in medicine. Medicine contains much sophisticated biology (of a restrictive kind, as we argue in many chapters). The average article presenting biomedical investigations has an advanced, technical level. This may invite the mistaken assumption that simple ideas and methods should always be suspect.

5.6. Fresh Inputs From Biology

The stage is now set for the strategy outlined in the Introduction. We indicated how the search for unconnected literatures can be rewarding (see the comments on Swanson's work). Our search concerning migraine yielded some interesting findings that connect items considered so far in new ways. For ease of recollection, a list of items from Section 3 should be helpful: spreading depression, vasoconstriction and vasodilatation, serotonin, inflammation, endothelium, endothelin-1, platelets, T-cells.

To begin with, we consider in greater detail the hypothesis of Swanson that magnesium is important in migraine. The hypothesis is embedded by him in a coherent set of relationships extracted from the literature. They include effects of magnesium on the following phenomena: vascular tone and reactivity (vasoconstriction and vasodilatation), spreading depression, aggregation of platelets, changes in serotonin levels and inflammation of blood vessels (inflammation of the endothelium). Swanson also suggests that magnesium plays a role in migraine induced by stress. This list is not complete. We omit items affecting migraine which we disregarded as we had to simplify. Swanson's result is well entrenched. The idea that migraine may represent a magnesium deficiency is supported by an impressive variety of indirect evidence.

We wonder how many key factors could be discovered in this way. Magnesium should be important, but many other factors could be equally important. We have anyhow found two additional factors that are hardly considered in the literature, to wit the hormone vasopressin and omega-3 fatty acids. We discuss them in this order. First, we return to some of the commonsensical ideas in the previous section to explain how we came to search for possible effects of vasopressin.

We argued that our eating and drinking habits affect the water balance in our bodies, and thereby our blood circulation. So these habits may be important in the pathogenesis of migraine. Vasopressin, or antidiuretic hormone (ADH), plays an important role in the water balance. It induces reabsorption of water in the kidney. Hence, if ADH is at a low level, urine production increases. ADH also plays a role in our becoming thirsty upon loss of water from our body. These effects are so well known, that it is natural to think of ADH as the hormone having this specific function. But hormones—and other substances in our bodies—are seldom if ever that specific, and interactions among hormones are pervasive. ADH has pronounced effects also on the balance of vasoconstriction and vasodilatation. Thus, it affects blood circulation in at least two ways, indirectly via an effect on water balance, and more directly by effects on blood vessels. Serotonin also affects, in a different way, vasoconstriction and vasodilatation. We would therefore expect that both substances may be implicated in migraine. Much research confirms that serotonin plays a role. A long chapter in Davidoff (2002) reviews all the evidence and mechanisms involved. Curiously, Davidoff does not mention vasopressin at all, and a search of Internet uncovers many articles on serotonin and migraine, and only a few articles on vasopressin and migraine. These articles, and a few sources providing indirect links, add up to the following picture.

Many forms of stress may provoke migraine attacks. Vasopressin plays a crucial role in the stress response and in depression associated with chronic stress, but its contribution has been largely neglected (Scott and Dinan, 1998). It is one of the hormones that counteract inflammatory responses (Chikanza and Grossman, 1998). Buschmann *et al.* (1996) observed increased platelet vasopressin receptors in migraine patients. Vasopressin subserves important vasomotor, antinociceptive, behaviour control, fluid and electrolyte balance, platelet aggregation and blood coagulation functions. As part of a complex homeostatic adjustment to stress and pain, the intricacies of vasopressin metabolism may have particular relevance to the pathophysiology of migraine (Gupta, 1997). High levels of vasopressin have been found in migraine patients, together with high levels of endothelin-1, a substance which has been implicated in migraine attacks (Hasselblatt *et al.*, 1999); vasopressin stimulates the synthesis of endothelin-1 in endothelial cells.

These results suggest that vasopressin may be as important as serotonin in migraine. The research community has been on the track of serotonin for a long time. Serotonin is mentioned, for example, in connection with psychiatric disorders, aggression and criminality. Indeed we feel tempted to see this as the great serotonin fashion. It is difficult to get specialised research from such one-sided tracks, however valuable they may be in some respects.

Our intention is not to replace the serotonin fashion by a vasopressin fashion. The point is rather that one-sidedness should be recognised for what it is. Also, our emphasis on vasopressin helps forge a connection with common sense and elementary biology, as we indicated in the previous section. Your eating and drinking habits influence vasopressin metabolism, and thereby should affect the chances that you may be prone to migraine. Our attitude would be that our primary interest, in science and in daily life, should be in these habits. If solutions for problems with migraine cannot be found there, it may be wise to resort to medications associated with sophisticated biomedicine. But this is unnecessary if solutions are to be found in more mundane ways.

The subject of food brings us to the second factor we like to consider, omega-3 fatty acids. First, we have some general considerations. Diet is a well-known item associated with migraine. Common wisdom has it that migraine may be provoked by particular foods such as cheese and chocolate. But this wisdom lacks the support of science. The passage from Davidoff that follows is revealing.

> Controlled data that might *prove* a relationship between diet and migraine attacks are meagre. ... Many patients have either placed themselves, or have been placed by physicians, on a restricted diet that has deprived them of chocolate, cheese, wine, and other foods all at one time without any attempt to determine that even one of the restricted items plays a role in the pathogenesis of their headache problem. The psychological stress of "cheating" on that diet, together with the fear that the food will cause a migraine, may be enough to trigger a migraine ... . The headache would then, of course, confirm the food as an offending trigger. [Many more pitfalls exist, and scientific research of the matter is difficult for methodological reasons.] (Davidoff, 2002: 95)

Our approach of diet and migraine is on the one hand more general than this: As indicated, we would focus primarily on eating and drinking in relation to patterns of daily activities. On the other hand, we have a more specific item. Research in many areas has shown that our average diet lacks adequate quantities of omega-3 polyunsaturated fatty acids (PUFAs). This appears to explain the commonness of many diseases, for example vascular diseases, autoimmune diseases and psychiatric disorders (see Chapters 7, 8 and 10). A reasonable *a priori* hypothesis would be that migraine is also affected by this.

Food supplements in the form of fish oil are rich in omega-3 PUFAs that are in short supply in our diet, notably eicosapentaenoic acid (EPA) and docosahexaenoic acid (DHA). EPA and DHA have therapeutic value in many diseases (for biochemical explanations, see Serhan and Oliw, 2001; Chapters 7, 8 and 10 provide many more references). We have done a search of the literature to find links between omega-3 acids and migraine. Few studies have been done on this in a direct way, but we have uncovered many indirect links.

Harel *et al.* (2002) obtained preliminary results suggesting that fish oil and also olive oil benefit adolescent migraine patients. But

Pradalier *et al.* (2001) found no significant effect in a large double-blind study, which disconfirmed previous studies with a more modest set-up. However, this finding concerns the last 4 weeks of a treatment period of 16 weeks. The entire treatment period yielded a significant difference suggesting that the omega-3 acids may be beneficial. More indirect evidence linking these acids with migraine takes many forms. We summarise a sample of recent evidence.

Omega-3 fatty acids affect the vascular system in many ways. Yamada *et al.* (1998) showed in experiments with rats that omega-3 acids, especially DHA, suppress platelet aggregation. EPA causes beneficial vasodilatation by several routes, some of which involve the endothelium (Engler *et al.*, 2000; Shimokawa, 2001). Jamin *et al.* (1999) found in experiments with cultured bovine endothelial cells that EPA decreases the release of endothelin-1. Furthermore, omega-3 acids have anti-inflammatory properties via changed quantities of immune system cells such as T-cells (Almallah *et al.*, 2000; Grimble, 2001; Terada *et al.*, 2001), and via a reduced adhesion of these cells to the endothelium (Mayer *et al.*, 2002; Grimm *et al.*, 2002; Sethi *et al.*, 2002).

The less recent overview by Smith (1992) is thought-provoking, as he provides an integrative account with elements that are seldom combined in the literature. He allots a central role to the immune system, arguing that pro-inflammatory substances from immune cells are released in migraine. Comorbidities of migraine with depression, infectious disease and trauma suggest as well that the immune system is impaired in migraine. According to Smith, prophylactic effects of fish oil (and primrose oil) also indicate that the immune system is involved in migraine, since omega-3 fatty acids in these oils counteract inflammation mediated by the immune responses. This integrative view is in keeping with later investigations.

We conjecture that comorbidity of migraine with psychiatric disorders may be due in part by fatty acid shortages in our diet, because fatty acid deficiencies appear to play a role in these disorders (see Chapter 10). Migraine is often associated with anxiety disorders and depression (see for example Guidetti *et al.*, 1998). Silberstein (2001) and Davidoff (2002: 20-22) note that the comorbidity of migraine and depression is bidirectional: each disorder increases the risk for developing the other affliction. This suggests that the two problems have a shared aetiology. We hypothesise that shortages of omega-3 fatty acids are an important shared factor.

In conclusion, the indirect links between the fatty acids and migraine are evidence that omega-3 deficiencies may be a significant causal factor in the aetiology of migraine.

5.7. Interlude: Neglected Disciplines

The new elements introduced in the previous section invite research with more emphasis on vasopressin in relation to common sense, and nutritional deficiencies. More generally, migraine research could benefit from disciplines which are seldom brought to bear on the subject.

First, approaches from psychoneuroimmunology may offer new insights. This discipline has focussed on all sorts of diseases and syndromes, for example cancer and autoimmune disorders. As far as we know, migraine has hardly been considered as a subject for research by representatives of this interdiscipline. It is indeed plausible that migraine should involve processes studied in psychoneuroimmunology, because stress ("psycho") influencing the nervous system ("neuro") causes inflammation ("immunology") that may provoke migraine. Furthermore, comorbidity with autoimmune disorders has been found in some cases of migraine. So it is reasonable to speculate that responses of the immune system to psychosocial triggers may contribute to migraine. Immune responses to stress may also expose migraine patients to toxins from invading pathogens that could provoke attacks (Covelli *et al.*, 1998).

Second, a discipline known as psychotherapy research should offer valuable insights (see Chapter 4). Davidoff insightfully portrays limitations of RCTs concerning placebos, but the subject merits much more scrutiny. Psychotherapy researchers have uncovered many subtle pitfalls shedding light on the comparative merits of drug treatments and psychotherapies. Conceivably, the balance of treatments for migraine may have to shift somewhat from drugs toward psychotherapy (Reid and McGrath, 1996; McGrath, 1999; Lake, 2001).

Third, research in the philosophy of biology, and other disciplines concerned with the role of genetics in biology and biomedicine, indicates that deep-seated forms of reductionism pervade much modern biomedicine (see Chapter 1, Appendix 2). We use here the term "reductionism" in the loose sense that low levels of organisation are overemphasised and over-represented. Davidoff's views show traces of this paradigm. For example, he departs from the fundamental distinction of primary causes in the aetiological sense, ultimately genetic factors, and triggers regarded as modifiers. As we have done throughout the book, we would defend here the view that factors in the two categories deserve the same "causal status," and we would plead for more research concerning higher levels of biological integration.

This view is defended also by Hellstrom (1999), who suggests that homeostatic balance is disturbed in migraine and many other disorders. Internal factors and external triggers may jointly shift the balance toward inappropriate activity and dysfunctional defence mechanisms. To understand what happens, we should primarily focus on high levels of physiological integration. Hellstrom's theory also implies that the existence of comorbidities calls for new approaches (see Section 6). Risk factors implicated in ischaemic heart disease, notably particular features of blood vessels, predispose toward other diseases including migraine. Thus, the study of shared aetiological factors may often be more fruitful than the study of countless idiosyncrasies of individual diseases. Diseases of the heart and the vascular system, for that matter, are affected by omega-3 fatty acid deficiencies, and treatment with these acids has positive effects in these conditions (for recent reviews, see Christensen and Schmidt, 2001; Kristensen *et al.*, 2001; Leaf, 2001; Nordoy *et al.*, 2001; see also Chapter 7.4). Thus, Hellstrom's theory may be united with our own suggestion that omega-3 shortages represent a shared aetiological factor of migraine and other diseases.

Fourth, philosophical reflection on the nature of scientific theories could be helpful. Davidoff shows on the one hand that migraine is a heterogeneous array of disorders, and that the value of theories about them is context-dependent in many ways. Yet, on the other hand, he appears to aim at a comprehensive theory of migraine which, he says, has yet to be developed. Considering the heterogeneity of migraine phenomena, we had better bite the bullet, and terminate endeavours to attain a comprehensive theory. Our aims should be modest, and we may have to be content with relatively specific theories, each applicable to a limited domain of migraine phenomena (for comments on the need of specificity, see Chapter 3, and also Van der Steen, 1993a; Burian *et al.*, 1996; Van der Steen, 2000a).

Fifth, as we argue in the next section, we should go back to history and retrieve from it valuable approaches and theories which got lost under the onslaught of molecular modernisation.

5.8. The Haystack in the Needle

Oliver Sacks, the neuroscientist, has published an impressive book about migraine in 1970, with an update in 1985. The book puts migraine in a broad context, with rich historical details. Much of what he has to say is still relevant today. We follow his lead to get migraine in the broad context it deserves, a context which has almost vanished from modern science.

Throughout the book, Sacks argues that migraine is at once a physical and an emotional phenomenon. Migraine attacks may also have or come to have symbolic value. Attempts to understand migraine without attending to experiential aspects are therefore futile. Sacks' overview of history is impressive and illuminating. Accounts of migraine span more than two millennia. The first modern treatise appeared three centuries ago. Many acute observers in the eighteenth century rightly made no difference between physical and emotional symptoms. Superb descriptions appeared with the opening of the nineteenth century. They had a vividness of description which has vanished from the medical literature. But most of these descriptions dwelt only on the physical side of migraine. Sacks maintains that the treatise of Liveing, which appeared in 1873, is a masterpiece which remains unsurpassed until the present day. Here is what he has to say about later developments:

> The present century [the previous one by now] has been characterized both by advances and retrogressions in its approach to migraine. The advances reflect sophistications of technique and quantitation, and the retrogressions represent the splitting and fracturing of the subject which appears inseparable from the specialisation of knowledge. By a historical irony, a real gain of knowledge and technical skill has been coupled with a real loss in general understanding. (Sacks, 1985: 7)

Sacks describes many cases in some detail. Let us look at one of them, case 62, and consider some implications.

> A 51-year old woman ... had suffered for more than twenty years with three somatic manifestations: common migraine, ulcerative colitis, and psoriasis. She would suffer for several months from one of these symptoms, before remitting and passing to another symptom. She was thus trapped within an endless malignant cycle. (Sacks, 1985: 48)

In modern scientific texts concerning migraine, descriptions of this kind are rare if they exist at all. How should we think about this woman? A study of her migraine alone would not get at the core of her condition. We have to discern the meaning of the entire cycle, and that is impossible without understanding her background and circumstances, and her emotional experiences.

Sacks' cases are richly varied, and they make clear that it is futile to search for *the* cause of migraine. We would add that, even if all migraine patients exhibited the same signs and symptoms, say, those of the case 62 woman, the search would be in vain. Whatever form it takes, the phenomenon of migraine comprises processes throughout the body. The nervous system is involved and the vascular system, and the immune system. We find effects at all levels of organisation from organs down to cells and molecules, and a rich variety of emotions is in play. Some diseases may allow of simplified descriptions with a limited number of aetiological factors, signs and symptoms. Migraine is not such a disease (for additional comments on this problem, see Chapter 2).

One way to describe the search for a single cause or a limited number of causes of migraine, would be to label it as looking for a needle in a haystack. But an even more appropriate metaphor would be that it is like looking for a haystack in a needle. It is unwise to attribute a rich variety of interconnected phenomena characterising a person to a restricted set of causes down to the molecular level. We have to apply stores of knowledge to patients. The search for the needle, or the haystack, tends to deteriorate into the application of patients to stores of knowledge, as we single out from their features those which happen to fit with bits of science we are interested in. This is not what Sacks is saying, but we think he would agree.

The problem we are envisaging applies to much science. At times, our interest in a theory justifies our abstracting from many features of phenomena. If we throw a stone out of the window to test Newton's laws, we may rightly disregard the colour it has, and many other features. Hypothetically, if we threw a woman out of the window, the same kind of reasoning would apply. But if we wish to understand women, this approach is unhelpful. Few genuine laws exist to help us understand the behaviour of women, or other living creatures.

All the subtheories about migraine apply usefully to many cases, seldom if ever to all cases. Considering any person with some pattern of migraine, we have to decide what knowledge is relevant in their case. The wise thing is to get to know much about the person and then to look for items from knowledge stores that fit the case at hand, not the other way round. However, this is not to say that generalities concerning migraine are entirely impossible. Sacks does formulate generalities, but they are open-textured. If details are filled in, they differ from person to person and from situation to situation.

Sacks regards migraine as a disorder of arousal. He argues that relatively stable, essential features may be recognised beneath all the variable and disjunctive components: alterations of conscious level, of muscular tonus, of sensory vigilance, and so forth (Sacks, 1985: 109). Notice that this kind of generality does not remotely resemble a quantitative law of nature. But it is clear enough, and it is useful. "Arousal" (also called "orientation") is a general concept from psychology, which has its uses also at the interface of biology and psychology.

Under stress, arousal may take the form of readiness to perform a flight-or-fight response, in animals and man. In principle, the response is functional as it can help us avoid an impending disaster, being eaten by a lion for example. Heightened awareness and vigilance under impending danger are associated with an altered state of the nervous system (activation of the sympathetic division of the autonomic nervous system), altered levels of many hormones, increased energy metabolism and much more.

As Sacks was writing his book, a common assumption was that responses to stress can be described with more detail in a general way. For example, the hormone cortisol has long been regarded as *the* stress hormone *par excellence*, its secretion being regulated by other known hormones. This assumption is no more. Recent textbooks will tell you that processes in stress responses are complex, and that their details depend on many contextual factors (see for example Moberg and Mench, 2000). But the general idea of stress inducing arousal and a flight-or-fight response is still valid. So is the assumption that the autonomic nervous system and many hormones (and the immune system) get into a different state under stress.

Animals and man may also respond in a different way to danger representing stress: immobilisation (freezing) is an alternative to the flight-or-fight response that may be functional, for example, if it prevents your being detected by an organism that would like to eat or shoot you.

These, then, are two major forms of responding to stress in the form of danger, which are found in much of the animal kingdom, however varied the forms they take may be in different organisms and different situations. Sacks argues that migraine belongs to the category of freezing responses. The responses may be highly functional biologically, as when you have been overloaded with impossible demands. Withdrawing somewhere with a headache where nobody is allowed to disturb you may then be a functional thing to do. It also allows you to recuperate, so that it may function like having a good sleep. However, the response may also become dysfunctional and grow out of proportions, if you are chronically unable to solve particular serious problems.

In this way, Sacks puts migraine in the context of a functional approach which characterises much biology. At the same time, the approach takes part in evolutionary thinking. The responses to stress occur throughout the animal kingdom, and we must have inherited them from our non-human ancestors. We agree that evolutionary thinking is relevant for the understanding of migraine. But Sacks' reasoning is somewhat simplistic. He does not mention the possibility that different species may have responses in common as a result of ecological convergence. In this case, different mechanisms serve the same function without an evolutionary connection. But we grant that human beings and mammals generally share many mechanisms underlying stress responses. Thus, Sacks' point may be well-taken after all. Anyhow, ecology and evolutionary biology are sorely missing in present-day approaches of migraine in biomedicine.

Functional approaches should be appropriate in many cases of migraine, but Sacks appears to overblow the matter somewhat. He argues that research on migraine should take place at the interface of biology and psychiatry. We would replace "psychiatry" by the more neutral descriptor "psychology." Sacks often searches for unconscious hidden motives that may provide a functional explanation of severe instances of migraine, although he grants that causal explanations may suffice in some cases. We would comment that dietary deficiencies may be responsible (causally, not functionally) for migraine and psychiatric disorders associated with it. If that were so in a particular case, then the search for adequate diets would be more appropriate than the search for hidden motives to explain headaches and abnormal behaviours.

The idea that arousal may be important in migraine has recently been taken up by the aid of electrophysiology in psychophysiological approaches (see for example Backer *et al.*, 2001; Davidoff, 2002: 153-155; De Tommaso *et al.*, 2002; Giffin and Kaube, 2002). Investigators have observed that, in periods between migraine attacks, patients show less habituation to visual stimuli than control persons. Habituation is the phenomenon that a repeated stimulus that first catches your attention fails to do so after a while. This finding fits well with the assumption that (some) persons with (particular forms of) migraine have a high level of arousal in normal situations. They may pay the price of attacks for this. The high arousal during an attack conduces to processes associated with a stress response. These habituation phenomena need not imply biological pathology. Conceivably, persons with a tendency to be very active in constructive ways, may as a result of this have "abnormal" patterns of habituation. That may provoke migraine in burdensome situations where high activity would be dysfunctional.

One item from Sacks' book is worth considering here as it

supports our own commonsensical approach described in Section 5 (Sacks, 1985: 29-31). He observes that the resolution of common migraine may proceed in three ways, as has been recognised since the seventeenth century. The migraine may exhaust itself and end in sleep, or it may gradually abate, or it may resolve by crisis, a sudden accession of physical or mental activity, which brings the attack to an end within minutes. Hard physical work, wrestling, or a violent rage are examples from the last category. Some of Sack's patients found out by themselves that this kind of thing works (for them). This is an example of engaging in activities that change the overall physiological state of the body. Sacks does not elaborate on the possibility that this amounts to a valuable therapy based on common sense and elementary biology. It is the kind of approach which we have defended in Section 5.

In closing, we mention an intriguing connection between migraine and visions of great mystics, described by Sacks in an appendix. The visions are interpreted in many different ways. Sacks notes that one of the greatest mystics, Hildegard of Bingen (who lived from 1098 to 1180), has left exquisite accounts and figures of her visions. He states that the accounts and figures were indisputably migrainous as they show all the characteristics of aura phenomena. We give no comments just now. In Chapter 12, we provide an extensive account of relations between religion, health and disease.

5.9. Conclusions

1. Research in biomedicine has virtually grown beyond comprehension. To counterbalance superspecialisation we have to build bridges between unconnected literatures.

2. Mainstream research on migraine has resulted in theories that are poorly integrated. This is not surprising, since migraine is a heterogeneous category of conditions. To understand migraine, we have to chart roles of blood circulation, the nervous system, hormones and the immune system. The roles of these systems are different in different patients.

3. The heterogeneity of migraine phenomena entails that randomised controlled trials (RCTs) do not have much clinical relevance in the search for migraine treatments.

4. Common sense and elementary biology may help us find new treatments of migraine.

5. The hormone vasopressin presumably plays an important role in migraine. Mainstream research has overlooked its significance.

6. The water balance of the body is related to blood circulation. Hence, accounting for the water balance should be important in migraine. The subject does hardly receive attention.

7. The existing ideas about food allergies in migraine may be inadequate as a possible dietary cause of migraine has been disregarded: a deficiency of omega-3 fatty acids.

8. The emphasis in research on migraine is overmuch on the cellular and the molecular level. Higher levels of physiological integration deserve more attention.

9. Functional and evolutionary approaches to be found in biology are almost lacking in biomedical research on migraine. They could lead to new, valuable approaches.

Chapter 6

Delusions of Psychiatry

6.1. Introduction

Your diet may determine whether you will stay sane or become mentally ill. Conceivably, for example, a vitamin deficiency may tip the balance toward abnormal mental states or behaviours. Psychiatrists know about this. In our country, and also in Germany for example, psychiatric patients are routinely screened for vitamin deficiencies that could explain their symptoms. Less well known in psychiatry, and in medicine, are deficiencies of particular fatty acids, omega-3 polyunsaturated fatty acids (PUFAs). These deficiencies are common and they contribute to many diseases and disorders. This is the main theme of Chapters 7, 8 and 10. In Chapter 10, we argue that existing approaches of mental illnesses (psychiatric disorders in another terminology) may not be optimal as effects of omega-3 deficiencies are underrated. In the present chapter, we introduce more fundamental problems with psychiatry.

Mental illnesses are elusive since relations between the mental and the physical have never been captured by a fully satisfactory scientific or philosophical theory (for references, see Chapter 12.1). The most sophisticated venture to find out about the relations, which draws on brain scan technology, is beset with many pitfalls (Uttal, 2001). It should not come as a surprise, then, that psychiatry has not come up with satisfactory theories of mental illness. It has many theories on offer, but no theory is without rivals that contradict it.

Psychiatrists have sought to steer away from this problem by theory-free classifications, particularly with recent versions of the Diagnostic and Statistical Manual of Mental Disorders, also known as the DSM. But the mere fact that much of the DSM is aligned to a medical model already reveals a profound theoretical commitment. It is anyhow impossible for classifications to be entirely theory-free. No philosopher of science would nowadays hold that we could ever do without theories.

The very attempt to approach reality without theories may make us lose touch with reality. The next section presents a telling example of this. We argue there that schizophrenia, a serious mental disorder with delusions, does not exist except as a fictitious thing in writings of psychiatrists. The idea that something in the real world corresponds with the notion of schizophrenia is a delusion. This is not to deny, though, that it may be wise for persons with serious delusions or other mental problems to consult a psychiatrist.

Good psychiatrists will readily grant that problems exist with their classifications and theories. Like the rest of us, they need a language to do their business. Words such as "schizophrenia" applied to some person may conveniently indicate that they are in a different category than, say, depressed persons. But the mere attribution of a DSM category to a person has no implications for disease status or treatment.

The current DSM version, DSM-IV (with DSM-IV-TR as the newest variant), follows a categorical rather than a dimensional approach: It construes mental disorders as more or less distinct entities rather than syndromes along a continuum of conditions. That is odd, because comorbidity, the presence of more than one disorder in a person, is very common in psychiatry (see, for example, Zuckerman, 1999). Comorbidity suggests that the disorders distinguished are artefacts with a limited basis in reality.

The DSM is also problematic as it fails to make a clear distinction between ordinary suffering and mental illnesses. Consider, for example, some of the diagnostic criteria for panic disorder without agoraphobia: (1) recurrent unexpected panic attacks, (2) at least one of the attacks has been followed by one month (or more) of one (or more) of the following: (a) persistent concern about having additional attacks, (b) worry about the implications of the attack or its consequences, (c) a significant change in behaviour related to the attacks.

We can imagine that a woman who has been subject to violent rape has these symptoms. That would be a natural response which need not deserve a mental illness label, however much she may need some form of treatment by a psychiatrist, a psychologist, or friends and neighbours. Likewise for persons who become depressed, say, after the loss of a spouse. The fact that a large proportion of the population satisfies DSM criteria indicates that the DSM approach invites medicalisation (for details, see Section 3).

An additional problem with the DSM is that its successive versions have been elaborated in undemocratic ways, with much influence from the pharmaceutical industry (for details, see Caplan, 1995; Kutchins and Kirk, 1997; Healy, 2002, reviewed in Section 3). The industry has a vested interest in categorisation, which helps in the marketing of drugs for allegedly specific conditions, and in a biological approach, which helps privilege medication over psychotherapy. Many psychiatrists may not wish to side with the industry, but in the present cultural climate they face a strong pressure in favour of medication.

Representatives of "biological psychiatry," an influential school nowadays, claim that mental illnesses are caused by biological abnormalities. This claim is often defended on the ground that they are associated with biological features. But to the extent that this is true, it does not prove much. The association does not by itself entail that the biological features regarded as "abnormal" represent biological *pathology* (see for example Fancher, 1995; Bowers, 1998: 175-178). For all we know, the biological features may represent normal responses to psychosocial adversity. Moreover, a biological pathology, if present, may have been caused by psychosocial adversity. In this case, the common view that biological pathology is a root cause with psychosocial factors in the role of modifiers, would be misplaced.

In the next section, which is based on a book by Boyle (2002), we explain why paradigms of biological psychiatry are problematic. In Section 3, we discuss additional criticism to be found in a book by Healy (2002), who also provides valuable information about overmedication and the role of the pharmaceutical industry in psychiatry. Section 4 provides additional comments on the current situation in psychiatry. A case study of anorexia nervosa in Section 5 illustrates potential uses of elementary biology in psychiatry. It is an illustrative example of *MSA* (missing stuffs and arrows, see Chapter 1): An old, valuable therapy that focuses on temperature regulation has long been disregarded by professionals concerned with anorexia. Finally, Section 6 puts psychiatry in a broad cultural context.

6.2. Getting Rid of Schizophrenia

Do mental illnesses result primarily from somatic impairments, particularly in structures or functions of the brain? Or do they represent responses to unfavourable social conditions? Both extreme views, and anything in between, keep being defended in confusing disputes.

The school of biological psychiatry puts much emphasis on genetic factors and brain abnormalities as causes of the disorders. Psychiatrists who belong to this school grant that other causes, for example psychosocial factors, play a role. But they generally regard them as modifiers or triggers that contribute to pathogenesis only if particular biological predispositions are present in the first place. Conversely, opponents of this view do not deny that biological factors are involved, but they regard other factors as causally more significant.

Which side should we take in this kind of controversy? An apparently reasonable response to this question goes as follows. In research on a particular disorder, say schizophrenia, we have to consider a great variety of possible causes. The results of our investigations will determine what causal factors are particularly significant. This kind of response assumes that the existence of the disorder is already known, and that new research adds to available knowledge. We claim with Boyle (2002) that this assumption is false since disorders such as schizophrenia do not exist. To avoid misunderstanding, we acknowledge that some persons with a diagnosis of schizophrenia suffer from a serious mental illness. Their illness is real enough. Our criticism concerns the nature of the diagnosis and its implications.

From some interpretations, not the one we have in mind, our claim that schizophrenia does not exist may sound like old news. Researchers in psychiatry would irrespective of their persuasion grant that in one sense schizophrenia, our example here, is not a well-defined disorder. No list exists of features that characterises all patients who suffer from "schizophrenia." So, if our claim were taken to mean that no such list exists, then it would be a platitude. Nor would the claim amount to much if it referred to the common idea that disorders have no existence apart from persons said to "have" them. Our claim is rather that the word "schizophrenia" as used in psychiatry is not connected with observable patterns in a scientifically meaningful way. Boyle (2002) has cogently defended this claim with many arguments and examples. We use her book as a guide.

Boyle reconstructs the entire history of the schizophrenia concept, and she provides a detailed analysis of all the relevant literature, particularly writings associated with successive versions of the DSM. We present her reconstruction in brief.

Schizophrenia, like other psychiatric disorders, is a syndrome, a clustering of symptoms and signs that tend to occur together at a greater than chance level. Syndrome names are abstractions inferred from observed patterns or regularities. To be useful scientifically, they have to allow predictions (Boyle, 2002: 11). The identification of syndromes is a two-stage process. If all goes well, symptoms as reported by patients allow the discovery of reliable signs that as antecedents of symptoms provide theoretical coherence (idem: 12). This has never been achieved in research on schizophrenia associated with the DSM. Indeed, researchers with leading roles in the construction of successive DSM versions often failed to make a proper distinction of symptoms and signs (idem: 89). This is a serious shortcoming, as we need signs in addition to symptoms to distinguish valid syndrome patterns from illusory patterns. Without some such distinction, sensible diagnoses are impossible for lack of genuine diagnostic criteria.

Diagnosis is a matching task. Medical practitioners aim to match physical phenomena displayed by patients with patterns already observed by researchers. This works well only if the patterns belong to theoretical frameworks inclusive of diagnostic criteria (idem: 82-83). Such frameworks have never materialised in psychiatry around the DSM. All the talk in psychiatry about validating diagnoses is therefore misleading. You can only validate a diagnosis of schizophrenia after prior validation of the concept of schizophrenia (idem: 90).

Contrary to a widespread misunderstanding, agreement among clinicians about diagnoses has no implications whatsoever for validity. Agreement represents reliability, which should not be confused with validity. With mere agreement masquerading as validity "researchers are 'discovering' what definitions clinicians use, or what instructions they follow, in applying 'schizophrenia' or other diagnostic labels, and then talking as if this told us something fundamental about 'schizophrenia' rather than something about clinicians" (idem: 91).

Boyle is aware that professional language in psychiatry is apparently at odds with her scathing comments. In DSM-III, the landmark edition of the DSM, diagnostic criteria were included. Afterwards, classifications and criteria have changed continually. Boyle comments that "although the process of producing diagnostic criteria is presented as one of continual progress, in practice it is one of trying to repair the shortcomings of previous versions of the DSM while avoiding a fundamental examination of the validity of its diagnostic concepts" (idem: 100). In a detailed analysis (idem: Chapter 5), she demonstrates that successive DSM versions represent a question-begging enterprise for lack of evidential links between 'schizophrenia' and regularities in the real world. This invites the question of how researchers were able to keep the enterprise alive over many years. Part of the answer would be that genetics appeared to provide researchers with a theoretical framework. Schizophrenia is said to have a genetic basis. However, as Boyle demonstrates in a separate chapter, research on the genetics of schizophrenia is flawed in many ways.

Twin studies are a case in point. Researchers commonly assume that schizophrenia must be determined in part by genetic factors, since concordance with respect to schizophrenia is much higher in identical twins than in non-identical twins. Twin studies proceed in stages.

> First, the sampling frame is selected, that is, the geographical and residential confines within which the

> 'schizophrenic' twins will be sought. Second, when this group has been selected, efforts are made to trace their co-twins. Third, the twin's zygosity [identical or non-identical] is investigated. Fourth (or concurrently) information is collected from the twins themselves and from other sources, and diagnoses are made. Fifth, concordance rates are calculated and interpreted. (Boyle, 2002: 155)

Boyle unearths serious errors in all the stages. Furthermore, the presentation of results in the literature is biased. Primary sources have been distorted in reviews of leading authorities. In the primary sources, the concordance rates for identical twins range from 69 per cent to naught (idem: 164). Such a thing is embarrassing. But the inconsistency can be dissolved by a disappearance trick, namely by broadening diagnostic criteria toward a "schizophrenia spectrum." In this way you can nicely increase concordance rates and decrease discrepancies. "As we can see [from a table], 'schizophrenia' can apparently be changed from a genetic to a non-genetic disorder [or the other way round] simply by altering the criteria used to infer it" (idem: 164).

> It will be recalled here that the variable cluster from which schizophrenia is inferred contains no sign, but only a number of ... behaviours called 'symptoms' and which have never been shown to be meaningfully related in ways required by the use of 'schizophrenia'. To use another analogy, if we call a pair of twins who share one or two of these 'symptoms', concordant for schizophrenia, it is almost like calling concordant for cancer a pair of twins where both report that they sometimes get headaches or feel nauseous. There is, in fact, no exact analogy for the absurdities of the schizophrenia spectrum; the major point to be made is that it is impossible to have 'lesser varieties' of a non-existent pattern. (Boyle, 2002: 166)

Concordance rates are further inflated by common, erroneous methods of calculation (idem: 166-168), and by overviews that omit disconfirming studies that lack case details while including confirming studies that also lack case details (idem: 169). Furthermore, other researchers have shown that the standard methods of calculating relative contributions of genetic and environmental factors to twin similarities are based on mistaken assumptions (see, for example, Mandler, 2001). Ideally, adoption studies of twins raised apart would have more evidential force, but the studies done until now do not satisfy elementary methodological requirements (Boyle, 2002; see also Joseph, 1999 and 2001, on twin adoption studies of schizophrenia and criminality, respectively). Considering the twin studies, Boyle misses one point which makes the situation even worse. Twin research deals with the population level. In itself, it has no implications for individual patients (for details, see Van der Steen, 1999a). For conclusions about individuals we need additional evidence from other sources. Boyle demonstrates that materials presented in the literature as additional evidence are nothing of the sort.

Studies known as genetic linkage studies have not produced convincing evidence either. Inconsistent results are the rule rather than the exception. “Finally, perhaps the most popular way of reconciling these conflicting results was to see them as confirming the idea that schizophrenia has many causes, or that only some types of schizophrenia are genetically determined” (Boyle, 2002: 201). This kind of ploy helps researchers to uphold cherished hypotheses against any adverse evidence.

After her devastating analyses of scientific research into schizophrenia, Boyle accounts for factors that keep “schizophrenia” alive. She notes that the concept of schizophrenia persists in the face of two major paradoxes (idem: 206). The first concerns the scientific status allotted to a concept against impressive evidence to the contrary. The second is “that it is not unusual for those who support the concept of schizophrenia to make statements which are, to put it bluntly, absurd but which are clearly intended or assumed to be sensible.” For example, leading researchers repeatedly state, on the one hand, that DSM criteria for inferring schizophrenia are “arbitrary” and, on the other hand, that they are “robustly valid” (see also comments of Ross and Pam, 1995, on articles in a leading journal of psychiatry). The “methodological innovations” ascribed to DSM-IV by its founding fathers “are frankly embarrassing, referring to processes so basic in science that it is rather like a modern chef announcing a methodological innovation in cooking—that you switch the oven on first.”

The researchers are still nowhere near evidence that “schizophrenia” is a valid concept, but they persist in doing highly technical research about the disorder. Many mechanisms contribute to this situation. One mechanism has to do with pattern recognition. Extensive research in psychology has demonstrated that human beings are prone to see a pattern where none exists.

> ... a spurious impression of co-occurrence of

> 'schizophrenic symptoms' might be fostered simply by the fact that several odd behaviors, even if they co-occur by chance, are more noticeable than only one. Thus, the psychiatric population who are, after all, those who have been noticed and brought to psychiatric attention, will by definition contain more cases of co-occurrence than of single disturbing behaviors. Although this process is likely to create a strong subjective impression of a pattern of co-occurrence where none exists, it might also be responsible for the creation of apparently significant statistical patterns. Indeed, Slade and Cooper [research published in 1979] reported that the correlation amongst 'symptoms' for those diagnosed as schizophrenic was no greater than the correlation found in a group of 'artificial' cases whose symptoms had been assigned randomly by the researchers. And if those brought to psychiatric attention already contain an excess of 'co-occurrences', then this impression is likely to be further strengthened by diagnostic practices. If psychiatrists regularly apply an official definition of 'schizophrenia', then inevitably a population will be created who seem to show a similar cluster of behaviors. (Boyle, 2002: 233-234)

Social forces help to keep this situation alive. The existence of "schizophrenia" and other psychiatric disorders as biological entities easily becomes desirable both for the professionals and for the general public (idem: 236-243). For professionals, the enduring conviction that mental illnesses or disorders exist in this way can serve as a substitute for research evidence. Also, schizophrenia conceived as illness helps to deflect criticism that psychiatrists act as agents of social control. Notably, the concept of schizophrenia has to remain vague and non-specific.

> This uncertainty has the triple advantage of retaining within psychiatry a 'disorder' which would have to be given over to neurology were it a *literal* brain disease; of creating an impression of important and progressive research whose future prospects are always bright and ensuring that it is never quite clear what does and does not serve as evidence for or against the concept. (Boyle, 2002: 237-238)

The public may benefit from biological conceptualisations as they may serve as exculpations. If the concept of schizophrenia as a brain disease were abandoned, then blame for disturbing behaviour would more readily accrue to the person or their family.

In the last chapter of her book, Boyle envisions alternative views. We have to grant that persons labelled as schizophrenic, or psychotic, exhibit "symptoms" such as delusions and hallucinations. But we should not take for granted that such symptoms always represent mental aberrations or, indeed, biological pathology. Studies of non-psychiatric groups demonstrate that between 10 and 40 per cent of people have experienced auditory or visual hallucinations (Boyle, 2002: 250-251; see also Coppock and Hopton, 2000: 119; Stephens and Graham, 2000). Hallucinations that take the form of hearing voices, for example, are common, but people in our culture who experience them may not readily report this, since voice hearing is not any more a done thing. You must be crazy if you experience it. In other cultures, though, your experiences may be taken to mean that far from being crazy, you have a gift that marks you as a person to be honoured.

Professionals in psychiatry confronted with hallucinations such as voice hearing in patients, have to decide whether a particular instance is pathological. Considering this, Boyle points out that many social and cultural factors may foster erroneous diagnoses that harm patients (idem: 265-267). The chances are that psychiatrists are more likely to come up with a biased judgment of pathology if imaginings are reported by someone who has already been devalued in some way, due to a low social status, poverty, or failures in social roles. The DSM itself would foster this kind of bias: It accommodates such sociocultural factors as criteria for inferring schizophrenia.

Psychiatry's dealings with delusions are as problematic as those concerning hallucinations. How are we to determine that a particular delusion represents pathology? Much research has shown that commonly used criteria are worthless. Should we regard odd beliefs as pathological if they are incompatible with beliefs widely held in the general population? Surely this will not do, since some implausible beliefs are widely held in the general population.

As dominant criteria are a failure, we are left with the idea that delusions are odd beliefs that are not culturally shared. This idea easily creates pernicious situations.

> [A serious problem with] the culturally understandability criterion for identifying delusions is that it implies that an observer's ability or willingness to

> understand how a belief system could have come about in terms of someone's life experiences or cultural background should serve as a criterion of whether the belief is a symptom of mental illness. The arrogance, absurdity and dangers of such a criterion can hardly be overstated. It implies, first, that psychiatrists (who are the defining observers in this context) could be omniscient, that they know or could know everything that could ever possibly be known about how environmental and personal factors interact to produce certain beliefs and are thus in a position to pronounce on when a belief falls outside this process; the criterion implies, second, that psychiatrists systematically and comprehensively assess the presence or absence of each of these factors and, third, having concluded that none is present, they are then entitled to infer mental illness or even brain disorder, even in the absence of any direct evidence of such abnormality. (Boyle, 2002: 273)

We conclude from Boyle's analysis of schizophrenia that psychiatry is in a position to heed a call for modesty.

6.3. Psychopharmacology: History With a Vengeance

Overmedication is common in psychiatry. Healy (2002) provides the most incisive account of the phenomenon. His book offers an extensive history of psychopharmacology, with rich details of interactions between psychiatry and the pharmaceutical industry, in a setting of politics and culture at large. The overall picture emerging from the book is appalling. Healy demonstrates that psychiatry has steadily deteriorated during the last few decades, while at the same time evolving into one of the most powerful forces shaping our society. But his analysis does not cover all psychiatry. Healy's target is biological psychiatry, particularly in the United States. Developments elsewhere have not been quite the same (see for example the volume edited by Gijswijt-Hofstra and Porter, 1998, which reviews the history of psychiatry in the United Kingdom and in The Netherlands). We concentrate on Healy's account since it deals with highly influential trends.

To start with, we review what Healy has to say about schizophrenia and the DSM. His account reinforces the view of Boyle that notions of schizophrenia associated with the DSM are deeply flawed. In one respect, Healy's analysis corrects views of Boyle. Healy is aware that some patients with "schizophrenia" suffer from a very serious illness, a point which is virtually disregarded by Boyle. He also shows that drug treatments have caused serious illness; this issue is outside the scope of the book by Boyle.

Most theoretical views of schizophrenia have centred on the distinction of positive symptoms and negative symptoms. The history of the distinction, as uncovered by Healy, demonstrates that we are now saddled with theoretical frameworks best regarded as myths, not science. The historical survey that follows is a summary of Healy's account (Healy, 2002: 265-270).

In the 1880s, Jackson introduced the idea that a disease may have negative and positive features. Bleuler used this idea in his account of schizophrenia in 1905. He distinguished primary negative features such as disturbance of thought processes resulting in incoherent language and action, from positive features such as delusions and hallucinations stemming from this primary loss.

From the 1960s onward, a confusing array of different conceptions emerged. Crow united these in the 1970s. He proposed that dopamine abnormalities cause positive schizophrenia (delusions, hallucinations), and that negative symptoms (flattening of personality, personal withdrawal, lack of volition, poverty of speech and thought) associated with changes in the brain develop later in some patients, possibly as a result of a virus infection. Crow had a flair for formulating an idea, and his view carried the day, even though all the substantial evidence at the time ran in the other direction (first negative features, then positive features). His view was in place by the time that tests were run with the drug clopazine. This drug appeared to have a beneficial effect on the negative features of schizophrenia. Both patients and clinicians were easily convinced that the drug was beneficial: The results were obvious.

However, the story of what was really going on is rather different. Effects of the drug had been compared with the effects of another drug, chlorpromazine, given in very large doses, in patients who had been on drug megadoses for a long time. The implications of this became clear only after many years:

> By 1990, however, research had made it seem quite possible that the only lesson to be learned ... was that administering clopazine was better than poisoning patients with drug cocktails or megadose therapies. ... The introduction of depot medications made it even more clear that some patients who were sitting at home

> quietly were in a state that was not, as first thought, the calm tranquillity of restored sanity but was rather a drug-induced withdrawal. (Healy, 2002: 268)

As laypersons and professionals began to realise that old drug treatments had caused a lot of harm, much pressure was exerted on the profession and on the industry to market better drugs. The result was a boom of so-called atypical antipsychotics. These drugs are still promoted with the argument that they should have less serious side effects than their predecessors, but this claim flies in the face of evidence (see Chapter 4.3). Within a couple of years, the market share of atypical antipsychotics rose to 60 per cent. The passage that follows explains how this could happen.

> The change stemmed from a mixture of wishful thinking and aggressive marketing. By the 1990s, pharmaceutical companies had discovered that patient activists were often the most effective lobbyists for the new treatments and they had allied themselves with some of the most aggressive patients groups [who had rightly fought horrendous megadose therapies in the 1960s]. (...)
>
> There were obvious difficulties for clinicians in accepting that even part of the benefits they were witnessing with the new drugs might stem from the fact that they were not now poisoning their patients to the same extent as previously. These difficulties led to a need for myths to disguise what was happening, and marketing campaigns for the new treatments that used the concept of negative schizophrenia vigorously provided the required mythologies. (Healy, 2002: 269-270)

Thus, we now are saddled with treatment-resistant schizophrenia transformed into a certain kind of negative schizophrenia created by the pharmaceutical industry. Instead, we should have retained older terms such as "catatonia," which do stand for non-artificial phenomena. Catatonia is a state which may last over long periods, in which patients are in a kind of stupor without any possibility of sensible contacts with other persons.

Healy's reconstruction of catatonia's history is illuminating (idem: 270-275). Nowadays, most psychiatrists assume that catatonia is a disease of the past as the advent of antipsychotics and social factors have led to early detection and prevention. However, in the 1950s, research already indicated that this could not be true. Some commonly used medications were then shown to induce catatonia-like phenomena. But this research was disregarded in mainstream psychiatry. In the 1960s, research led to the recognition of so-called neuroleptic malignant syndrome (NMS), a dangerous condition caused by neuroleptics (antipsychotics). Subsequently, researchers in the 1980s noted striking similarities between NMS and catatonia. They also found out that the two conditions respond to similar treatments, for example barbiturates. Indeed, the effects of barbiturates had been outlined decades before. Also, the researchers discovered that catatonia had not disappeared at all. Psychiatrists were assuming this, but neurologists knew better. In the 1990s, catatonia-like symptoms appeared to occur with rates of 5 to 10 per cent in some general hospital psychiatric units.

How could such a situation arise? During a long period, much evidence existed that catatonia had remained a not uncommon condition. But the evidence was ignored by most researchers and practitioners in psychiatry. Healy states that "the answer has to be that no company stood to make money out of encouraging clinicians to recognise catatonia. The patent on lorazepam, which was remarkably effective in treating the condition, had expired" (idem: 273). The industry did militate against market development profiles that would dismantle the schizophrenia monolith by the recognition of catatonia. The appalling conclusion has to be that knowledge which could save lives has become ineffectual as it did not have the backing of the pharmaceutical companies; we note, though, that catatonia is recognised in The Netherlands, lorazepam being the treatment of choice.

The case of catatonia illustrates the influence of the industry on the classification, the diagnosis, and the treatment of psychiatric disorders. It is by no means the only case. Here is an additional example. Moynihan (2003) reports in a recent article that the pharmaceutical company Pfizer has managed to create female sexual dysfunction as a new disease to be treated with drugs marketed by the company.

The industry has influenced theories of aetiology and pathogenesis as well. The so-called transmethylation hypothesis of schizophrenia is an example (Healy, 2002: 182-192). In the 1950s and the 1960s, the transmethylation hypothesis, actually a collection of related hypotheses, received much attention. The hypothesis was supported by a well-confirmed theory which suggested that particular treatments, notably with vitamin B3, should be beneficial. Positive results were obtained with this treatment by Hoffer and others (for details, see also Hoffer, 1998, who later moved to alternative medicine in the form of orthomolecular psychiatry). Critics were unable afterwards to confirm this, but those in favour of the hypothesis and allied therapies countered that the critics were being influenced by the pharmaceutical industry and organisations with vested interests. Interest in the hypothesis faded away in the course of the 1960s, and it was never resurrected. But adverse evidence was not the cause of its demise. It was to be replaced by the (by now discredited) dopamine hypothesis of schizophrenia. Here is how Healy describes the replacement:

> The transmethylation hypotheses proposed a pathological mechanism as the source of the clinical features of psychosis. From that kind of theory, logical therapeutic strategies can be derived. The dopamine hypothesis of schizophrenia, in contrast, argued backward from the efficacy of the treatment to what might be the cause of the disorder. That made little more sense than arguing that because aspirin was useful in treating rheumatoid arthritis there must be some kind of aspirin deficiency implicated in rheumatoid arthritis. Yet, despite its weakness, the dopamine hypothesis of schizophrenia was successfully used by the pharmaceutical industry to sell drugs. (Healy, 2002: 191)

In other words, we have here a promising theory that was overshadowed by a bad theory as the bad theory was financially profitable.

The evidence reviewed so far demonstrates that external forces caused a steady deterioration of theories and allied practices in psychiatry. This looks like an amazing development, since increasingly strict guidelines regulating scientific methods of drug testing saw the light in the period considered here. A reasonable assumption would be that the enforcement of such guidelines should lead to better theories and treatments, but developments were in the opposite direction. To explain this apparent paradox, we have to scrutinise the methods. We review here Healy's analysis of randomised controlled trials (RCTs; see Chapter 4.2 for details), which are regarded as the most powerful tool of research on treatment effects.

The history of RCTs is complex. Before the 1960s, regulation of drug marketing and drug use did not require evidence of efficacy and safety. In many cases, the effects of drugs were so conspicuous, that demonstration of efficacy was superfluous. But the crisis of thalidomide, a drug that caused serious birth defects, was conducive to a dramatic change in health care in the United States (idem: 366-369). Drug therapies suddenly became "risky," and in 1962 amendments to the 1938 Food and Drugs Act sought to channel drug development and drug availability towards acceptable risks of treatment offset by benefits. Companies were encouraged to develop drugs targeted at specific disease indications, and drugs were to be available only by prescription. Also, the amendments introduced RCTs, but inclusion of placebos became obligatory much later, by the mid-1980s.

The amendments put a premium on categorical rather than dimensional models of disease, by analogy with the exemplar of bacterial infections. Categorical models treat diseases as distinct entities with clear defining features, whereas dimensional models recognise continua and overlaps (see also the comments in the previous section). Beforehand, the emphasis in the mental health arena had been on a dimensional approach. The change toward a categorical approach has had unfortunate effects in psychiatry (idem: 284). RCTs work best with homogeneous samples of patients. The use of such samples led to artificial fitting of patients into categories of the DSM. The use of the categories easily evoked the illusion that drugs tested with positive results have "specific" effects.

Classifications of drugs in psychiatry boosted this image. Thus, the name "antipsychotic" evokes the idea of a drug with specific effects on psychosis. In fact, the classifications, for example antidepressants *versus* antipsychotics, are suspect as they are often at odds with science. "The concepts of an antipsychotic and an antidepressant are neither chemical nor pharmacological. They are social constructs" (idem: 228). Some labels without scientific merit were indeed used as slogans as they have a high marketing value (for example atypicality, as in atypical antipsychotics; idem: 254). The idea of specificity was anyhow suspect as the drug companies also managed to market products with alleged benefits for a variety of conditions.

RCTs in psychiatry also had devastating effects on the role of evidence. Clinical judgment became suspect. The companies explicitly recruited patient samples of convenience. No guarantee existed that the results obtained should be valid in real-life situations. Healy argues that the reformers ultimately produced the opposite of what they set out to achieve. A continual interaction between companies and regulators ultimately led to massive overmedication with bad drugs (idem: 306-309 and 371-374).

Some placebo-controlled trials of drugs were done in the period from 1960 to 1984, but most trials were restricted to comparison of new and old drugs. The comparisons generally failed to show that any of the drugs actually worked. Placebo controls in regulatory studies were not instituted until the mid-1980s, initially to the dismay of the industry. This caused a setback in the development and marketing of new psychotropic drugs, the more so as dangerous side effects were being recognised by now, with legal liabilities for the industry.

This situation appears to have fostered the licensing of Prozac by the FDA in 1987. New drugs were needed after all. Studies including a placebo were done with Prozac, but the overall evidence in its favour was weak. By this time, the evidence that counted belonged to the pharmaceutical industry. "Throughout the 1990s, a succession of drugs with minimal effects on depression was licensed, in some cases with only two out of six trials showing a superiority to a placebo, with any trials that failed to show a differentiation from a placebo being termed failed trials" (idem: 308; for additional comments and references, see Chapters 4.3 and 10.2).

Healy argues that the enormous increase in the apparent frequency of depressive disorders and other psychiatric conditions during the 1990s is directly attributable to intensive marketing of antidepressives such as selective serotonin re-uptake inhibitors (SSRIs) and other drugs by the pharmaceutical industry. The industry gathers evidence favourable to its own interests. It has a strong influence on clinicians and on the public at large. "Increases in the incidence of conditions by a thousand-fold [as in obsessive-compulsive disorder] do not appear to surprise clinicians and the public has had a newly minted biobabble substituted for the psychobabble prevalent during much of the century" (idem: 373).

We are also being cheated by the active suppression of evidence. "SSRIs can be shown to 'work' through the use of clinician-based disease-specific rating scales. But when patient-based non-specific rating scales, such as quality of life instruments, have been used in trials, the drugs cannot be shown to work, and this information has not seen the light of the day" (idem: 373).

Remarkably, one recent development has been toward the use of drugs without the "benefit" of RCTs. In the late 1990s, anticonvulsant drugs were used increasingly to treat bipolar mood disorders, without RCT demonstrations of efficacy (idem: 321). RCTs are highly impracticable in this case, since it is difficult to assess a condition that cycles from one pole to its opposite. Thousands of patients would in this case have to be studied over many years. Clinical judgment is thus the best option. Cases such as this one suggest that "RCT-derived evidence affects clinical practice primarily in cases where trials fail to provide evidence of efficacy. ... Perhaps the most important use of such evidence today ... is its rhetorical use by governments, third-party payers, or drug companies attempting to gain control of a market" (idem: 322).

However, the RCT paradigm still holds sway, and psychiatry, like all medicine, is now infused with the idea that we have managed to develop an ideal of "Evidence-Based Medicine," with RCTs in a prominent position. Healy's views of this idea are well expressed by the heading of one section (idem: 320-327): Evidence-*Biased* Medicine. In psychiatry, the idea has led to extensive medicalisation of ordinary problems of living (idem: 348-351; for additional sources and comments, see Chapter 10.2).

By the end of the 1990s, the control of behaviour extended well beyond the management of people with genuine disorders. The mental health service has developed into a mental health industry. In the United States, a quarter to a third of the population with depressive symptoms or distress are thought to need treatment. More than ever before, treatment is driven by a concern for enforcing behavioural norms.

RCTs and quantitative instruments for symptom assessment, for example the so-called Hamilton Depression Rating Scale (HDRS), have the function of detecting small differences between patients and nonpatients (the point is here that statistical significance need not entail clinical relevance; see also Chapters 4.3, 9.4 and 10.2). Decades ago, such approaches were unnecessary, as conditions such as catatonia could be treated with dramatically effective drugs. No quantitative approach was needed then to obtain convincing evidence.

By now, we have massive medication. Numerous children with problem behaviours are forced to take Ritalin, a drug with a pharmacological profile resembling that of cocaine (idem: 173). Antidepressants are prescribed in large quantities on the basis of flimsy evidence (for additional sources, see Chapters 4.3 and 10.2).

Healy notes that young generations of clinicians are hardly able to stand outside technologies such as RCTs and the HDRS. These technologies help demonstrate minimal effects in clinical trials. But the effects have no basis any more in clinical practice. Clinical knowledge, the essential basis for a humane treatment of patients, has been overrun by the myth that quantitative methods promoted by moneymakers should pave the way toward well-being.

This is an extreme verdict. We concur with it—with some caveats. Healy's comments apply to derailed implementations of quantitative Evidence-Based Medicine. It is true that informed clinical judgments should be superior to the derailments. But these judgments have limitations also (see Chapter 4.4). We need both quantitative and qualitative methods (for additional comments, see Chapter 9). Current Evidence-Based Medicine is one-sided as a theory, and its applications are often unsound. But this does not mean that we have to discard it lock, stock and barrel. We have to recognise its limitations and improve on the current situation (for a balanced account, see Goodman, 2003).

Evidence thrives in a great variety of locations. Let us visit as many locations as we can.

6.4. Addenda From Miscellaneous Sources

The analyses by Boyle and Healy summarised in Sections 2 and 3, and the sources they mention, suffice to show that dominant approaches in biological psychiatry are inadequate, that many drug treatments are ineffectual and dangerous, and that overmedication has become disastrous (see also Chapters 4.3 and 10.2).

Meanwhile, we see no signs that methodological criticism is taken seriously by staunch defenders of biological psychiatry. For example, recent volumes on the genetics of psychiatric disorders exhibit all the trends criticised by Boyle (see section 2), the old prophecy that future findings are going to improve on present inadequacies (see the volume edited by McGuffin *et al.*, 2002), and the old promise that sophisticated techniques make such findings feasible (see the volume edited by Leboyer and Bellevier, 2003). A representative volume edited by Helzer and Hudziak (2002) aims to pave the way for a new, improved edition of the DSM, without visible changes in the style of research. The views expressed by Kendell (2002) in the first chapter of the book are characteristic.

A positive point in Kendell's account is the admission that categorical approaches may have to be replaced by dimensional approaches (see Sections 2 and 3). But in other respects, it is all old wine in new bottles. Kendell emphasises that great progress has been made in improving the reliability of diagnoses based on the DSM, but he has to grant that validity is still a major problem. Boyle made the point that this situation has existed for a long time, and that it reveals a fundamental inadequacy of DSM classification and research associated with it (see Section 2). The endless succession of putative improvements is worthless as long as invalid concepts are the foundation of the entire undertaking.

Kendell has remarks about this which have been heard for a long time. "It is important to appreciate that failures to demonstrate the presence of a valid boundary ... never prove that there is no boundary to be found" (Kendell, 2002: 12). This, of course, is true by definition. But Kendell does not address a pressing question: Whose is the burden of proof? After all the DSM years, the burden should not be with the critics, but with those who defend the classification.

"We already have strong evidence that genetic factors make a major contribution to a wide range of mental disorders ..." [but the situation is difficult because many genes are typically involved] (idem: 13). True enough: All features of organisms are influenced by genetic factors and environmental factors. But that is trivial. As Boyle (and many others before her; see her references) has shown, non-trivial claims in the literature are methodologically suspect. Nowhere does Kendell mention the most acute criticism of genetic analyses in biological psychiatry.

Kendell repeatedly remarks that success will be forthcoming in the long run. It all takes time, because "the human brain is an infinitely more complex machine with a much wider range of functions than the heart, the kidney, or the liver" (idem: 13). This is one of the ploys mentioned by Boyle. The current failures are transformed into a promise of success. The ploy is prophecy, not science.

Kendell also has an interesting comment on the commonness of psychiatric disorders:

> The fact that some psychiatric disorders have a surprisingly high prevalence in the general population does not necessarily mean that they have been inappropriately defined. Some people do regard it as absurd that at any given time 10%-15% of the population is suffering from a mental disorder and that nearly 30% may do so in the course of a year; however, I believe that this reaction is related to the stigma associated with mental illness. (...) It was demonstrated long ago, much to everyone's surprise at that time, that most people have troublesome physical symptoms most of the time. (...) If physical disorders are so common ... there is no reason why psychiatric disorders should not be equally common, and it would be a mistake, both scientifically and politically, to change our definitions in order to reduce their apparent prevalence. (Kendell, 2002: 6)

This passage is out of all bounds. Kendell admits that the validity of the DSM is poor. Hence, the mistake has been that we have adopted it at all. It is indeed true that we should not change DSM definitions to reduce the prevalence of disorders. That would amount to rejecting them for the wrong reasons. But critics would reject them for the right reasons. They would argue that the definitions are demonstrably inadequate, and that applying them has resulted in an inflation of prevalence. The comparison with physical disorders is also fallacious. The structure of Kendell's argument is as follows: "*X* is common, therefore the thesis that *Y* is not common is false." If you wish, you can argue in this way that uncommon things do not exist.

The volume in which Kendell's contribution appeared (Helzer and Hudziak, 2002) was published by the American Psychopathological Association (APA), which has close affiliations with research geared to the DSM. The other contributions to the volume also bear the imprint of this. We get much biology, with psychology at best geared to biology, and the DSM recognised as amenable to improvement, not rejection. A volume published by the American Psychological Association (Beutler and Malik, 2002) also concerns the need to change the DSM. In this volume, the emphases are different. The contributors argue that we have to live now with improved versions of the DSM, while searching for alternatives.

The neuroscientist LeDoux (2002) does not belong to the DSM circuit, but he has affinities with biological psychiatry. His view of developments in biological psychiatry is captured by the passage that follows.

> Regardless of how one feels about the biological orientation of psychiatry today (and it has many critics), two facts must be acknowledged. The essence of who we are is encoded in our brains, and brain changes account for the alterations of thought, mood, and behavior that occur in mental illness. (...)
>
> Biological psychiatry was founded on, and still largely adheres to, the assumption that mental disorders are due to chemical imbalances in the brain. The brain, in this view, is like a delicate soup. To maintain its characteristics, just the right mix of key ingredients is required.
>
> [Meanwhile we have learned:] Mental states are not represented by molecules alone, or even by a mix of molecules. ... they are instead accounted for by information processing within and between synaptically connected neural circuits. Chemicals participate in synaptic transmission [and the circuits determine mental states].
>
> Biological psychiatrists do realize that circuits are significant, and it's not out of ignorance that they adhere to the soup model. They would love to have smart drugs ... that ... would go straight to the circuits

> that underlie a particular disorder and avoid all others. With this sort of drug, dreaded side effects would be eliminated. [But our present knowledge is not yet sufficient to realise this.] Although not all the pieces of the puzzle are in place today, research efforts are under way to obtain the information that would make this possible. (LeDoux, 2002: 260-262)

Again we are facing prophecy. This particular prophecy is flatly contradicted by biology. The idea that circuits or sets of circuits in the brain exist that operate in isolation, without influencing each other, would make for an odd organism, a dead organism actually.

We feel more sympathy for the views of Heinrichs (2001), who provides a detailed, excellent overview of research into schizophrenia, with an emphasis on biological psychiatry. He observes that findings concerning the aetiology and the pathology of schizophrenia never apply to all patients. This is a sign that existing approaches have fundamental shortcomings:

> Perhaps the kind of illness that produces the findings reviewed in this book is an illness that cannot be accommodated within current views of brain function, behavior, and neurological disease. What if the findings that have accumulated with respect to schizophrenia violate or contradict in a basic way the current neuroscience approach to mental illness? The synthesis of evidence shows that no abnormality in brain or behavior can be found in all people with a schizophrenia diagnosis. Yet within the spectrum of evidence, cognitive abnormalities occur with substantially greater prevalence than do biological abnormalities. Indeed, more than a third of the biological research literatures are not only very modest in strength but unstable and unreliable as well. Perhaps this situation means something important about the adequacy of neuroscience thought in relation to the schizophrenia puzzle. Perhaps it also means something important about the adequacy of attempts to understand the mind in neurological terms. (Heinrichs, 2001: 270)

In Heinrichs' book, prophecy-like elements or claims with the flavour of advocacy are nowhere to be found. His knowledge of the literature is extensive, and his sources are up-to-date. His survey confirms the view of Boyle that biological psychiatry cannot deliver the goods it has been promising for a long time. Heinrichs (2001: 272) aptly notes: "The problem is that neuroscience still uses the old medical paradigm and lacks a theory and a model of how biological events become mental events that become schizophrenia."

This is also the message which Uttal (2001) defends in a book-length analysis of modern neuro-imaging, a collection of sophisticated techniques to scan the body. Neuro-imaging has recently become a great success in medicine, as it allows an accurate localisation of lesions, major lesions, that is. The techniques have also become a research tool in biological psychiatry. Uttal's message is not good news for those who enthusiastically apply the new technology to the investigation of subtle changes in the brain allegedly characterising particular mental illnesses. To begin with, he shows by an extensive historical overview that instability has always characterised classifications of mental functions in psychology. Modern classifications in cognitive psychology and cognitive neuroscience are no exceptions. Alter a classification, and you will get different results from imaging studies. Furthermore, the results of such studies depend strongly on the values of parameters that need to be set to get the imaging process going. Alter the value of a parameter, and you get different results. Uttal also analyses methodological problems with the interpretation of results. All the problems uncovered by him are seldom considered in research articles that make use of the techniques.

If we add to this what we have learned from Boyle and Healy, we get a bleak picture. We can compare patients with controls in some imaging study. But as the classification of mental disorders is problematic, we cannot be sure that our standard of comparison is appropriate. Next, the persons have to be investigated in the artificial setting of laboratories, where their behaviour will differ from that in real life situations. We control the experimental conditions, so that our results will not apply to situations in which conditions are different. Then we choose to focus on particular variables that interest us. On top of this, we get all the limitations catalogued by Uttal. Any results obtained in this way are meaningless unless very large differences between patients and controls are found. But if such differences materialise, we are not allowed to infer general claims from our results.

Our analyses so far were limited to biological psychiatry around the DSM, mostly research done in the United States. But the DSM is not the only game in town, and research in other countries has often taken productive routes disregarded by biological psychiatrists in the United States. In Germany, for example, many researchers use classifications that may not invite harsh verdicts like the DSM does. At least one classification of psychiatric disorders in Germany, developed by Leonhard in the 1980s and 1990s, is not as arbitrary as the DSM, because it keeps reliability and validity apart.

Franzek and Beckmann (1999), who follow Leonhard's approach, argue convincingly that his classification, unlike the DSM, has a promising level of validity. A twin study undertaken by them confirms Leonhard's view that "schizophrenia" as defined in the DSM is a mixture of disorders with different genetic backgrounds and different aetiologies (but the authors do not recognise all the limitations of twin studies mentioned in Section 2). We do not present Leonhard's classification here, because it is only one among many existing alternatives to the DSM, all of them disregarded in mainstream biological psychiatry.

One interesting item associated with the Leonhard classification deserves to be noted here. In Section 3, we mentioned the odd history of catatonia as described by Healy: Catatonia seemed to decline over the years, but this was to a large extent a medication artefact wrought by the pharmaceutical industry. Researchers working in the Leonhard tradition have recently shown that catatonia is more common according to Leonhard's criteria than according to DSM criteria (Stompe *et al.*, 2002). According to them, the prevalence of catatonia has been deflated by a combination of classification artefacts and medication artefacts.

6.5. Anorexia Nervosa: Lessons From Biology

We have deliberately paid the most attention to schizophrenia. Common opinion has it that this severe disorder is the best paradigm of biological roots in mental illnesses. As problems exist with research on the biology of schizophrenia, we can reasonable assume that biological views of less severe mental illnesses are also problematic. We have indeed uncovered a great many problems with existing views of schizophrenia in biological psychiatry. Thus, we can safely assume that this can be generalised to other mental illnesses.

A rejection of current biological psychiatry does not imply that biology has nothing to tell us about mental illnesses. In Chapter 10 we argue, for example, that dietary deficiencies may cause biological abnormalities resulting in mental illness. The case study of anorexia nervosa in the present section also concerns diet, though not in the same way. We show by way of this case study that elementary biology can sometimes be more helpful in psychiatry than all the sophisticated biology which now dominates research.

Anorexia is associated with ideals of physical beauty. Different cultures have different ideals, and ideals in any particular culture have a habit of changing over time. In Western countries, ideals concerning body weight and shape, of women particularly, have increasingly shifted toward thinness. This is presumably one of the factors that explain why anorexia nervosa has become a noticeable psychiatric disorder during the last few decades. Anorexia occurs predominantly in women. It is associated with dieting as patients tend to starve themselves. But dieting is not the sole factor in the aetiological story. The rest of the story is complicated and not entirely clear (for a survey, see Polivy and Herman, 2002). Also unclear is what therapies offer the best opportunities for a cure (see Kaplan, 2002, about psychotherapies, and Zhu and Walsh, 2002, about medications).

Anorexia has some remarkable biological features that help to explain why it tends to resist treatment. Anorexics often complain of feeling cold and have body temperatures below normal. This is not entirely a matter of poor abilities to retain heat due to loss of body fat. Additionally, the energy metabolism of the patients is comparatively low (Russell *et al.*, 2001). This impairs their temperature regulation. After a meal, they may sweat and feel hot instead of cold. The food is then to a large extent "wasted" as heat. This may be a functional response that helps body temperatures go back to normal, but it thwarts weight gain.

Therapies have focussed on the problems with eating in disregard of the problems with thermoregulation. There is an important exception, though. Blumberg (2002) notes that Gull (1874) long ago emphasised the need to supply external heat to the patients when they eat. "Such treatments fell into disfavour during the twentieth century with the uninhibited growth of the psychopathology industry" (Blumberg, 2002: 195). Fortunately, Blumberg notes, control of the patient's thermal environment is now making its comeback as a therapeutic resource: Berg and Södersten (1998) report impressive success rates with anorexics for a therapy in the spirit of Gull.

The example of anorexia uncovers valuable resources from elementary biology. It has much in common with our approach of migraine in the previous chapter. The issue was there that regulation of the water balance in the body may be expected to influence blood circulation and thereby migraine. In the large literature about migraine, we did not find a single reference to this aspect of physiology. Examples such as these suggest that the emphasis in current biomedicine is overmuch on sophisticated molecular biology, at the cost of the good old biology which recognised the importance of physiological regulation at higher levels of organisation. This kind of biology should be honoured in psychiatry. In biological psychiatry, it has virtually disappeared.

In closing, we have another interesting point about anorexia. Healy (2002: 360-361), in considering eating disorders, observes that all theories have neglected a development that occurred in parallel with eating disorders: the introduction of weighing scales in the 1870s. The subsequent growth in the weighing scale industry parallels the growth in the frequency of anorexia.

6.6. The Fate of Psychiatry

Our analysis results in a negative picture of psychiatry. The DSM, the most widely used classification of psychiatric disorders, is for many reasons an unacceptable edifice. Its successive versions fail to show signs of improvement. The role of biological abnormalities in mental illnesses is overvalued on a basis of poor science. It is true that abnormalities or injuries of the brain may result in impaired mental functions. Strokes and brain tumours are obvious examples. We also know that the dementias are caused by brain pathology. The biological study of such conditions is an uncontroversial element of neuropsychology (see, for example, Zillmer and Spiers, 2001). A variety of the disorders studied by psychiatry also have a known organic cause (for a survey, see the textbook by Lishman, 1997). We are not concerned here with such conditions. The great majority of mental illnesses are in a different category. Convincing evidence that they represent pathology in the biological sense has not been forthcoming. Nonetheless, they are often brought under the aegis of biology. As well, problems of living are being medicalised into mental illnesses. The pharmaceutical industry has created much medicalisation and the overmedication associated with it. Psychotherapies are an obvious candidate to help us counter some of these trends. But as we saw in Chapter 4.4, these therapies are often as problematic as drug therapies.

Our approach has been one-sided, as we have concentrated on biological psychiatry associated with the DSM. Alternative approaches come in many different, unconnected kinds. We review a limited sample of approaches to indicate what changes of emphasis could help us improve on current biological psychiatry.

The example of anorexia in the previous section is a good starter. If it is true that temperature regulation goes awry in anorexia patients, and that manipulation of ambient temperature is a promising therapy, then we have here an example of biology fruitfully contributing to psychiatry. Indeed, in opposing biological psychiatry, we do not mean to oppose biology in psychiatry. The point is to extend the fashionable study of genes and brains with research on higher levels of physiological integration.

The possible association between anorexia and weighing scales illustrates that biology, however broadly conceived, does not suffice as a scientific base of medicine. At times, we can only understand manifestations of disease if we are willing to move beyond the traditional boundaries of biomedicine. We already made this point in Chapter 3, with examples revealing the significance of structural violence and poverty in biomedical theorising (for more comments on the issue of boundaries, see Chapters 11 and 12).

An old tradition in the philosophy of medicine does plead for a replacement of the biomedical model by a biopsychosocial model (Engel, 1977 and 1981). However, the biopsychosocial model is methodologically unacceptable (Van der Steen and Thung, 1988: 192-195). It regards the body as the locus of biological features, and restricts the environment to psychosocial features. In this way ecology falls by the wayside. Thus, influences of diet on health and disease are easily missed (see Chapters 7-10). While rightly emphasising the importance of psychological and social factors, proponents of biopsychosocial approaches do us a disservice by deflecting the study of disease from effects of the physical and the biological environment. Unfortunately, the approach is alive and well. Kiesler (1999) has recently applied it to psychiatry. He demonstrates that biological, psychological and social theories of mental illness are all inadequate, and then elaborates an integrative theory which accommodates elements from these theories. But the biology in his theory is still the old, one-sided biology of the biomedical model.

Functional approaches of behaviour are an ingredient of psychotherapies assimilated by psychiatry, but they are missing in biological psychiatry. In biology and in psychology, functional explanations have a legitimate place alongside causal explanations. In Chapter 5.9, we argued that functional explanations may help us understand particular cases of migraine. For some persons, migraine may be a functional response which helps them recuperate from extreme stress. This must not be generalised, though. If a dietary deficiency is implicated in migraine, a causal explanation of attacks may be more appropriate than a functional explanation. It all depends on the person and the circumstances.

This situation also applies to mental illnesses. Bolton and Hill (1996) have developed a philosophical theory which makes room for functional as well as causal approaches in psychiatry. They defend the view that intentional causation and non-intentional causation are different processes. The technical details, which are difficult and controversial, do not concern us here. On the basis of abstract philosophy, the authors present concrete examples of intentional causation that illustrate the value of functional analyses. Thus, they argue that hallucination and delusion in psychosis may be part of a coping strategy that benefits patients (Bolton and Hill, 1996: Chapters 8 and 9).

> Intentionality in psychological processes entails the experience of continuity, coherence, and efficacy. Where the environment is reasonably benign and decipherable, and where action is possible and effective, these experiences are supported. Threats arising either internally or externally or in combination, may be countered via mechanisms that entail sacrifice in order to restore meaning and action. The sacrifice of accuracy of perception [as in delusions] in the pursuit of clarity and action may be a particular (but not exclusive) schizophrenic strategy. (Bolton and Hill, 1996: 341)

The functional interpretation of delusions in the passage quoted may well apply to some patients. But psychosis may also be induced by poisoning, or by dietary deficiencies. A causal approach would be more fitting than a functional approach when such factors play a significant role.

Explanations that see in hallucinations and delusions a coping strategy, will have to allot a significant role to unconscious processes. Theorising about such processes is hampered by much confusion about the meaning of "unconscious." Orbach (1995) distinguishes five major psychotherapeutic models of the unconscious: the psychoanalytic approach, the humanist approach, an approach centring on dissociation, the cognitive approach, and an approach postulating mental incongruence. He also distinguishes four views of relationships between the models: they represent different theories of the unconscious, or they amount to the same thing and only differ in terminology, or they refer to different processes and problems, or they reflect processes associated with different personality structures.

We do not want to opt for any of these possibilities. Orbach's survey illustrates that theorising about the *mental* in mental illness is now a quagmire (see also Section 4.4). As long as this situation exists, we like to follow a commonsensical approach. The analysis of the situation in the United Kingdom by Coppock and Hopton (2000) has a refreshing flavour of common sense.

Coppock and Hopton (2000: 1) begin their analysis by noting: "Since the late 1950s, one of the most striking features of the published literature on mental health is the plethora of books and articles which challenge the assumptions of mainstream medical psychiatry and clinical psychology." But the critiques are seldom brought together, and the critics do not acknowledge ideas of reformers within mainstream psychiatry which are similar to their own. It is true that medical psychiatry is implicated in policing and socio-political control mechanisms, and that it adheres to unproven ideologies which contradict the experiences of distressed persons. Thus, the critics must be taken seriously. But many of them ignore evidence against their own hypotheses (idem: 5).

The emphasis since the 1950s has been on drug treatments and biological psychiatry. "What does give cause for concern ... is the subtle operation of a hierarchy of ideologies which seems to privilege discourses which incorporate biological psychiatry over all competing discourses" (idem: 165). Most approaches of mental illness emphasise individual pathology. That is deplorable. "However, there are situations where the causes of a person's distress are beyond their control and where conventional therapeutic responses are of limited value. For example, the problem may be inability to get access to material resources, daily experience of discrimination, social isolation or even a fundamental lack of self-confidence" (idem: 176-177). For such problems, the authors envisage therapeutic communities as a possible solution that requires a reform of mental health care. "If mental health care in the community is to become a reality, mental health professionals will need to undertake community development work" (idem: 179).

This strikes at the heart of the matter. Psychiatry is being saddled with social ills of our society. Its professionals may try to avoid this and stay within restricted boundaries in conformity with science. If they do that, then they are easily saddled with intellectual ills of our society: Modern science has become overly materialistic and it has divorced itself from the humanities. We cannot understand human flourishing and human suffering from within the confines of modern science. But psychiatry is being forced to the make believe that such a thing should be possible. Add to this the common belief that psychology and social science should be subordinate to biology, and we get biological psychiatry as a natural outcome.

It is possible in principle to change the intellectual outlook, but that is a tough undertaking against the flow of funding from sponsors with vested interests. Any change of outlook with less emphasis on biology and on medication would be a great good, but it would not be enough. Existing social ills call for a new culture in which being in distress has ceased to be the measure of being human. As long as we are far removed from this utopian ideal, psychiatry is likely to remain in an unenviable position.

6.7. Conclusions

1. Existing classifications of psychiatric disorders, particularly successive versions of the Diagnostic and Statistical Manual of Mental Disorders (DSM), are out of touch with reality. For example, the concept of schizophrenia is almost useless. The symptoms of patients may be real enough, but combinations of symptoms listed in the DSM are artificial. The prevalence of symptoms such as hallucinations in the population at large is high. As the prevalence of hallucinations tends to be underestimated, medicalisation is a continual threat.

2. The pharmaceutical industry contributes to medicalisation and overmedication in psychiatry. Biological psychiatry also contributes to this trend. Its approaches are one-sided as it overestimates the role of biological pathology in mental illnesses, as often as not on the basis of poor science.

3. Quantitative methods, notably randomised controlled trials (RCTs), have a restricted value in the assessment of psychotropic drugs. Outcomes of RCTs have to be supplemented with evidence from other sources.

4. Elementary biology may have useful roles to play in psychiatry. For example, simple measures that compensate for impaired temperature regulation in anorexia nervosa are a promising therapy.

5. Biological psychiatry has many shortcomings, but this does not imply that we have to dispense with biology in psychiatry. Potentially valuable contributions from biological science are now disregarded as genes and brains are at the centre of research. We need more ecological thinking in psychiatry, and more emphasis on high levels of physiological integration and on functional approaches. But biology is not enough, as psychiatry is forced to deal with social sources of distress beyond the grasp of biology.

Chapter 7

Fatty Acids, Health, and Disease

7.1. Introduction

None of us can do without food for a long time. Whatever our disposition and character, the need to have meals, preferably several times a day, is one of the things that unites us.

Everybody knows that the quantity and the quality of the things we consume affect health and disease in many ways. Yet most medical research articles on particular diseases do not consider possible influences of diet. The review of literature in the present chapter demonstrates that this is a deplorable oversight (for additional information, see Chapters 8 and 10). The quality of diets in Western countries has been declining during the last century. Most notably, deficiencies of particular fatty acids (omega-3 polyunsaturated fatty acids, PUFAs) contribute to many chronic diseases and psychiatric disorders.

You will not find much about the deficiencies in the average textbook about nutrition. This is a serious lacuna. We do not mean to imply here that texts without lacunae should be feasible. The simple line of reasoning that follows indicates that such a thing is impossible.

Let us focus on the fate in your body of carbohydrates from a dinner you consumed. Textbooks in biology tell you that they are converted into comparatively small molecules, sugars for example. These may be used immediately as a source of energy for many processes in the body and activities of the body—the person—as a whole. But part of the sugars will be stored after being recombined into larger molecules, with glycogen as a storage compound, and fat as an additional storage facility in the presence of excess caloric intake. Upon a need of energy mobilisation, the glycogen may be broken down again to provide raw materials that are a source of energy.

Textbooks offer diagrams with names of substances interconnected by arrows that represent causal pathways, to make the biochemical fundamentals of metabolism visible. For example, a diagram concerning the metabolism of glucose may present many "metabolic pathways" indicating relationships with other domains of metabolism.

Glycogen and glucose, a sugar, are connected by arrows in either direction; from glucose you have a route to interconnected organic acids that jointly form the so-called Krebs cycle; another route goes from glucose to fatty acids that are components of fats, and so forth. Added to the diagram may be names of enzymes associated with the arrows. Enzymes are substances that enhance the chemical conversions represented by the arrows.

Such diagrams are always incomplete as substances are missing. Also, the arrows to and from substances are restricted to chemical transformations regarded as significant in the context of interest. Such simplifications serve us well. Without them, we would be overwhelmed by unmanageable quantities of information. However, the missing stuffs and arrows are also a potential source of dysfunctional one-sidedness. For reference, we have introduced the abbreviation *MSA* for them (see Chapter 1). We also use the expression in a more general way, for missing things and / or connections between them.

It is all too easy to see the diagrams as representations of an objective reality, while they are actually artificial means to represent a miniscule fraction of interconnected processes in our bodies. To the extent that we are not aware of *MSA*, we may inappropriately restrict medical research and medical treatments to routines and recipes that happen to flow from information in diagrams and other artificial sources (see also Chapter 2, for similar comments on classification and diagnosis).

The existing emphasis in biomedical research on genetics and molecular biology invites *MSA* in the broadest possible sense. Temple (2002), in a review of nutrition and disease, presents an apt characterisation of this one-sidedness:

> The human body may be likened to a black box of immense complexity. Various factors enter the black box and the end result is health or disease. Ideally, one may wish for a proper understanding of the inner working of the black box. In practice, however, identifying the relation between incoming factors (diet, life style, and the environment) and resulting health and disease is sufficient for an understanding of how to prevent disease. Based on this analogy medical research has been divided into two types: complex and simple.
>
> *Complex research*
>
> This type of research consists of studies of

disease mechanisms. The large majority of studies in such areas as biochemistry, physiology, and molecular genetics are examples of complex research. This type of research appeals to the human sense of curiosity. However, disease mechanisms usually prove to be so complex that we enter an almost never-ending quest for clear answers. This type of research is also referred to as *mechanistic* or *reductionist* research.

Simple research

This type of research comprises those types of study where the results indicate what factors cause or prevent disease. Of course, the research itself may not be simple. The main forms of simple research are epidemiologic studies (ecologic, case-control, and cohort studies), intervention trials in humans, and analogous studies on animals. Biochemical and physiological measurements may be included with simple research if they are clear indicators of disease risk. (Temple, 2002: 343)

Temple argues that, in the area of diet and disease, simple research has generated the most important information, whereas most of the funding goes to complex research. We argue that this imbalance has resulted in erroneous views of diet. Inadequate dietary recommendations concerning fats and fatty acids have been around for a long time. Evidence of widespread fatty acid deficiencies existed, but it was ignored. This is a deplorable example of selective perception, indeed, selective non-perception of valuable insights. Examples in the next section concerning diet and health illustrate how the established order resists new insights. The remaining sections review effects of fatty acid deficiencies in a great variety of diseases. Chapters 8 and 10 provide additional information about the deficiencies in particular diseases and disorders. Chapter 8 deals with rheumatoid arthritis and peptic ulcer disease, Chapter 10 with psychiatric disorders.

7.2. Doing Away With the Cholesterol Myth

Erasmus (1993) has since the 1980s campaigned for changes in the composition of existing diets in developed countries, which are unhealthy overall. He argues convincingly that modern diets cause health problems as they have an inadequate fatty acid composition owing to food processing and other factors. We discuss this subject in the next section, on the basis of more recent literature. From Erasmus' book we take views on another fascinating subject, cholesterol and heart disease (Chapters 12 and 71 of his book).

Cholesterol, like all the fats and fat-components discussed in this chapter, belongs to the lipids, a group of substances that dissolve in organic solvents. It plays vital roles in our body. It helps regulating the fluidity of cell membranes, and it is an important precursor of some hormones. But it has also been branded as a substance that becomes dangerous if we have too much of it.

Here is the bad news as told over many years by the medical community, the pharmaceutical industry and health care organisations. Cholesterol, if present in the blood in large quantities, is a major cause of atherosclerosis, the deposition of plaques in blood vessels that may ultimately cause heart attacks, or strokes, or kidney failure. The original story has become more refined over the years. Cholesterol takes different forms, only some of which are considered dangerous. To avoid the danger, we must take care to use unsaturated fatty acids in our diet. Also, if blood measurements indicate that we are in the danger zone, we had better use medications that restore the cholesterol balance. Before turning to details of this story, we outline an alternative story reported by Erasmus.

Rath, together with Pauling, winner of two unshared Nobel prizes, also controversial as a founder of orthomolecular medicine, have in the early 1990s turned the common medical theory about atherosclerosis on its head by arguing that lack of vitamin C is the culprit. Unlike most animals, we cannot make this vitamin from glucose. For an adequate intake we have to consume many fresh greens and fruits. Nowadays, methods of food processing and food storage in "civilised" societies result in diets with vitamin C shortages.

Rath and Pauling argued that atherosclerosis is caused by a particular protein (a different one than the culprit seen at the time by the medical community), and that vitamin C decreases the availability of this protein in our blood. Erasmus notes that vitamin C cannot be the whole answer for problems with blood vessels. Many other nutrients are involved. The important point is that viable alternatives for the medical atherosclerosis dogma are visible only if we are aware of *MSA* (see the previous section).

Rath and Pauling first submitted their article with the vitamin C story to a prestigious journal, which accepted it and subsequently refused it (a highly unusual thing), and then published it in a little known journal.

Erasmus identifies economic and political influences in the ensuing controversy over atherosclerosis:

> Those whose income depends on treating diseases of our heart and arteries by less effective or ineffective means, who profit from the fact that sickness is better business than health, and whose priorities place profit before truth, cure, care, and life stand to lose much from a solution to the puzzle of human cardiovascular disease ... .
>
> This political and economic controversy is part of an age-old battle between natural healer and drug pusher. (Erasmus, 1993: 72)

There are those in the medical community who would not respond kindly to such statements. They would be right in so far as Erasmus formulates his point in an overly general way on the verge of unjustified mud slinging. Over and above being an eminent professional, Erasmus is an engaged advocate, and we can understand the expression of his concern. Barring his general phrasing, his point is well taken (see Chapters 6, 8 and 10).

Ravnskov (2000) has devoted an entire book to the issue. His analysis of policies and literature demonstrates that selective reporting favoured the cholesterol myth over opposing views, that conclusions and recommendations in publications endorsing the myth were often at variance with the data, that trials with drug treatments or diet treatments aiming to reduce risks of heart disease via effects on cholesterol were often flawed, and so forth.

Stoll (2001), in an excellent book about fatty acids, health and disease, also argues that we need to get rid of the cholesterol myth. Like Erasmus, he allots a central role to nutrition. In Chapter 2 of his book, which has much on cholesterol, Stoll begins his tale as follows.

> One of the great medical myths of the past fifty years has been the notion that fats (more properly called lipids) are evil. Of course, like all other enduring myths, there is a grain of truth at the core. Literally thousands of studies over the past half century have traced high-fat diets to increased risk of heart disease. The most famous of these, the Framington Heart Study, followed a representative sample of 5,209 adults in Framingham, Massachusetts, to examine the circumstances and risk

> factors associated with heart disease. The Framington study was an epidemiological study designed to learn how those who develop cardiovascular diseases differed from those who remain free of the diseases over a long period of time. (...)
>
> Along with such culprits as smoking and sedentary lifestyle, the Framington scientists found danger in diets high in fat. (Stoll, 2001: 27)

The scientists paid much attention to saturated fat and cholesterol as culprits. They overlooked the effects of particular polyunsaturated fatty acids (PUFAs; see the next section).

With regard to cholesterol, the Framington Heart Study has led to a view which has remained in circulation for a long time. Cholesterol needs carriers called lipoproteins for transportation in the blood. These come in two kinds, the high-density-lipoproteins (HDLs) and the low-density lipoproteins (LDLs), which after being bound to cholesterol yield "good" cholesterol and "bad" cholesterol, respectively. The bad cholesterol was assumed to be responsible for the cholesterol-containing plaques in atherosclerosis.

Recent research has shown that cholesterol biochemistry is more complex than this, but the idea that it plays a role in atherosclerosis and diseases associated with it, has remained in force. Furthermore, a dominant theme is still that unsaturated fatty acids, both in monounsaturated and in polyunsaturated form, help to achieve a countervailing metabolic force. Stoll notes that this is still the official view of the American Heart Association (AHA).

Both Framington Heart Study researchers and the AHA have failed to make a distinction between omega-3 PUFAs and omega-6 acids PUFAs (see the next section). Once you get the picture, you will see that this is an example of unacceptable *MSA* (see Section 1). The distinction makes nonsense of the entire cholesterol story and all the simplified tales about unsaturated fats. The next section introduces the distinction in more detail.

7.3. Introducing Omega-3 Fatty Acids

Ever eat purslane? Perhaps you do not even know this vegetable. In The Netherlands, where we live, it used to be eaten quite often, but its popularity is on the decline. We are told that it is even less popular in the United States. Yet, conceivably, if our ancestors in prehistoric times had not cherished it, we would not have passed into existence. Neither would we be here, if ancestors of ours in more remote periods had not relied on diets with several essential components that are now sorely missing (for details, see the next section).

Physicians in the past knew that purslane has healing powers in addition to nutritive value (Stoll, 2001: 52). In ancient Greece, Hippocratic physicians used it to treat headaches, stomach and intestinal ills, heart problems, inflammatory problems, and shortness of breath. In this respect, their wisdom may surpass that of some present-day physicians, who prescribe drugs in large quantities against such conditions (see Chapter 8).

Purslane is a rich source of alpha-linolenic acid (LNA; also abbreviated as ALA), a fatty acid that belongs to the so-called omega-3 group of the PUFAs (Simopoulos and Salem, 1986; Simopoulos *et al.*, 1992; Simopoulos *et al.*, 1995). The average diet in "civilised" countries is poor in omega-3 PUFAs. This is a cause for concern, because we need these fatty acids to stay healthy. The existing shortages are implicated in many diseases. According to most investigators, we also need in our diet a proper balance of omega-3 PUFAs and PUFAs in another category, omega-6. In common diets, omega-3 PUFAs in addition to being in short supply, are overshadowed by omega-6 PUFAs. For the record, we note that Horrobin (2000 and 2002), who has done much research on the role of fatty acids in schizophrenia, does not endorse the theory that relatively high levels of omega-6 PUFAs are harmful.

For our ancestors, the omega-3 PUFAs must have been abundantly available (for details concerning their food, see the next section). That is why their bodies needed no enzymes to produce them from other foodstuffs. They may have lost genes coding for the enzymes, or they never acquired them. Anyhow, they must have benefited from omega-3 PUFAs in their diet over a very long period. We still do not have the enzymes, whereas many other animals have them. More accurately, LNA is a so-called essential nutrient that must be in our food as we have no enzyme to produce it. Our bodies do have enzymes to convert LNA into docosahexaenoic acid (DHA) and eicosapentaenoic acid (EPA), but only in amounts that do not meet our requirements.

The shortage of omega-3 PUFAs in our diet is disastrous. Before describing the causes and the consequences in more detail, we briefly explain why the acids are important (for details, see Simopoulos, 1991 and 1999; Stoll, 2001; Calder, 2002). Once eaten and absorbed by the body, omega-3 and omega-6 PUFAs go through conversions along two pathways. First, they become incorporated into cell membranes and, second, they are converted into hormone-like compounds called eicosanoids, prostaglandins among them. Omega-3 PUFAs make membranes more fluid. Thus, they have a profound influence on our entire biochemistry and physiology. That alone explains why shortages of these acids may result in many different diseases. The PUFAs are crucially important in the functioning of the immune system. Just like they have key roles in chemical signalling, so do they influence the behaviour of many different cell types subserving immune responses (see for example Grimm *et al.*, 2002; Singh *et al.*, 2002). We do not describe processes at the cellular level in the present chapter, because they are different in different diseases. Particular examples of omega-3 PUFAs influencing cellular immunity are to be found in Chapters 5.6 (migraine), 8.4 (autoimmune diseases and gastric ulcers) and 10.4 (mental illnesses).

The eicosanoid pathway is complex. Basically, omega-6 PUFAs produce inflammatory eicosanoids, whereas omega-3 PUFAs have the opposite effect. But this is not to imply that we can miss the omega-6 PUFAs. These acids, too, have important functions. But they need to be kept in check by the omega-3 PUFAs (Simopoulos, 2002b; Calder and Grimble, 2002). If the balance is not right, this may again result in all sorts of diseases (but Horrobin does not agree with this; see Horrobin, 2000; Horrobin *et al.*, 2002).

All these things are only now in the process of being slowly recognised by the medical community at large. Yet they have been known for many years (see Clandinin and Jumpsen, 1997, for a general survey and references, and the next section for additional details and references). Recognition of the scientific evidence is slowed down by an inadequate organisation of nutrition research, food inspection and regulation.

> In many Western countries, including the United States and the United Kingdom, nutrition research is either shared by the Departments of Health and Agriculture (USA) or is carried out by the Department of Agriculture (UK). Neither of these situations is satisfactory, and having the Department of Agriculture in charge represents a conflict of interest as shown by the problems in 'mad cow' disease. (Simopoulos, 2001b)

Worse still, the food industry has managed to "infiltrate" the World Health Organisation (WHO) and committees of the Food and Agricultural Organisation (FAO), as Boseley (2003) reports in the *Guardian*. These situations have resulted in unscientific dietary recommendations for the prevention of cardiovascular diseases and cancers, for example. Inadequate diets are to a large extent responsible for the high prevalence of these diseases in Western countries (see the next section).

Conflicts of interest at the bottom of official dietary guidelines are documented extensively by Nestle (2002). She presents much evidence to show that food companies have a far-reaching influence on politics in the United States. As a result of this, official guidelines derive from politics as much as from science. Food supplements pose particular problems since the law is less strict with the marketing of supplements than with drugs. Pharmaceutical companies are allowed to market drugs only after positive effects have been obtained with randomised controlled trials (RCTs). By no means does this guarantee that all is well with the drug market (see Chapter 4.3). Guidelines notwithstanding, the pharmaceutical industry has managed to flood the market with large quantities of drugs that do not serve public health. Food companies are likewise engaged in floodings. Their situation is less difficult as they do not have to reckon with RCTs. But regulations exist to prevent misleading advertising. After much political haggling, existing regulations have recently been weakened so much that the food companies seldom face problems with the authorities. Existing guidelines are anyway hard to implement. Hence, numerous food supplements and enriched foods are being propagated with health claims that are problematic from a scientific point of view.

This situation puts us in a complicated position as we advocate the use of omega-3 PUFAs as food supplements. As we are writing this, the industry is promoting these PUFAs, and enriched foods containing them are now being marketed. But we are not aware that the industry is using arguments such as ours.

Nestle has an interesting point about omega-3 PUFAs:

> The FDA's ongoing struggles to maintain scientific integrity in the face of pressures from the industry, Congress, the courts and, presumably, the public, are best illustrated by its dealings with requests for supplement health claims. In October 2000, the agency issued a "letter" announcing a new dimension in health claims—a "qualified" claim in which supplement producers could link omega-3 fatty acids (the "good" fats from fish oil and some plants) to reduced risk of coronary heart disease. In a 36-page review of research on omega-3 fats and health, the FDA concluded that use of such supplements was safe and lawful, but that the weight of the evidence required the label to include this

> qualification: "The scientific evidence about whether omega-3 fatty acids may reduce the risk of coronary heart disease (CHD) is suggestive, but not conclusive. Studies in the general population have looked at diets containing fish and it is not known whether diets or omega-3 fatty acids in fish may have a possible effect on a reduced risk of CHD. It is not known what effect omega-3 fatty acids may or may not have on risk of CHD in the general population."
>
> From a scientific standpoint, this statement is a balanced summary of the current state of knowledge. From a marketing standpoint, however, it is hard to imagine how it might fit on a supplement label, let alone whether anyone might read or understand it. Perhaps for this reason, toward the end of 2000 the FDA gave a million dollars to the Institute of Medicine to develop a scientific framework to help the agency evaluate the role of dietary supplements in health. (Nestle, 2002: 269-270)

We agree with most of Nestle's views, but considering the omega-3 PUFAs we disagree with her. Like the FDA, she presumably assumes that RCTs should be the paramount source of evidence. On this assumption, the case in favour of omega-3 PUFAs is admittedly not very strong. But additional sources of scientific evidence exist, many of them poorly known or even unknown in disciplines concerned with health care. We argue that, overall, the evidence compellingly shows that omega-3 deficiencies are common, and that omega-3 PUFAs added to our diet benefit health.

Omega-3 PUFAs play distinct roles in the brain, which is special biochemically. The passage of substances from blood to brain tissue is limited by the so-called blood-brain barrier. Many factors influence the passage from blood to brain of PUFAs, some of which are needed by the brain in great quantities. The PUFAs must pass the membranes of the barrier, and the membranes themselves need omega-3 PUFAs to allow the passage (see the overview by Banks *et al.*, 1997).

It should not come as a surprise, then, that omega-3 PUFAs have special significance for psychiatric disorders. Stoll (2001) has extensively investigated effects of omega-3 PUFAs on depression and bipolar disorder, with promising results. The group of Horrobin and Peet has developed a new theory of schizophrenia based on the role of fatty acids in membranes (see for example Horrobin, 1997; Peet *et al.*, 2001; Horrobin *et al.*, 2002; Peet and Horrobin, 2002). The relations between PUFAs and psychiatric disorders are discussed in greater detail, with more references, in Chapter 10.

Holman (1997) has investigated possible deficiencies of PUFAs in somatic diseases. He observed that shortages of omega-3 acids lead to severe conditions in many diseases, for example neurological diseases such as multiple sclerosis (MS), Huntington's disease, anorexia nervosa, and diseases with impairment of the immune system such as Crohn's disease and sepsis. More recent surveys also indicate that omega-3 acids play a role in many diseases, especially neurological diseases (Katz *et al.*, 2001) and autoimmune diseases (Simopoulos, 2002a; see also Chapter 8).

Effects of omega-3 PUFAs in Huntington's disease deserve special consideration, as they may have far-reaching implications. The disease is characterised by involuntary movements and progressive dementia. It mostly has a late onset, during middle age, and ends in sudden death after about ten years. It is a paradigm example of a serious genetic disease with a known mode of inheritance. Puri *et al.* (2002) treated patients suffering from the disease either with ethyl-EPA, a derivative of one of the omega-3 fatty acids, or with a placebo. The results were spectacular. After 6 months the patients receiving ethyl-EPA had improved whereas the patients on placebo had deteriorated. Brain scans showed progressive brain atrophy in the patients on placebo, and the reverse process in the patients on ethyl-EPA. This result is significant as a counterbalance to naive views about genetic determination. The notion of genetic determination is meaningless without reference to the environment, since all features of organisms depend on genetic and environmental factors. A disease may be "genetic" in one environment, and "non-genetic" in a different environment. Thus, if our diets became more appropriate, we could witness drastic changes in the genetics of health and disease. By implication, the existing emphasis on genetics in research may yield one-sided views of aetiology. This is not to deny that genetic factors are important. Genetic differences between persons are indeed associated with differences in their responses to nutrients in general and omega-3 PUFAs in particular (Simopoulos, 1995a and 1995b; Grimble, 2001).

Holman (1997) has an apt characterisation of the dietary deficiencies:

> We should take measures to ensure that adequate levels of omega-3 polyunsaturated acids are present in the diets of our populations. This can be done most easily by shifting our use of edible oils from

> omega-6 oils to the more balanced omega-3 + omega-6 oils, such as soy oil, canola oil, and flax oil. [Oils should not be hydrogenated. Increasing the content of fish in our diet would help.] Perhaps our traditional foods should be re-examined. In both hemispheres of this world, the major populations still produce beef as a principle source of protein. However, in industrialized countries, our management of these creatures has in recent decades concentrated on producing animals for marbled beef, produced in feedlots by overfeeding with crops containing linoleic acid as the principle polyunsaturated acid, and starch as the principle source of calories. The bovine species was originally a grass eater, and grass contains linolenic acid. Cows are what they eat, too. If their feed does not contain adequate sources of the precursor, linolenic acid, their muscles will not contain a normal quota of long-chain omega-3 PUFA. (Holman, 1997: 177-178)

Ever eat hamburgers? Perhaps it is time to replace them by purslane and all that.

7.4. Learning From the Past

Eaton and Konner (1985) and Simopoulos (1991, 1997, 1999 and 2001a) have in their reviews put the omega-3 story in an impressive broad context. They put together evidence from many areas: evolutionary biology, the history and prehistory of agriculture, epidemiology applied to cross-country comparisons, experimental studies with animals concerning dietary deficiencies, and long-term studies of medical dietary treatments. The emphasis in their work is on cardiovascular disease and cancer. Informative literature on the role of diet, including omega-3 PUFAs, in these diseases has been appearing since the 1950s, but some significant messages in this literature were ignored in mainstream medicine.

The bearing of evolutionary theory on aging is one among many interesting themes in Eaton and Konner (1985). Common wisdom has it that natural selection has not eliminated diseases of old age, as it fosters reproductive survival, not survival as such. Since lifespans of human beings have increased owing to better food and hygiene, they paid a price for it in the form of late onset cardiovascular diseases and cancers. Eaton and Konner unearth literature, in part dating from the 1950s (!) that casts doubts on this view. Young people in the Western world often have asymptomatic forms of these conditions, and members of technologically primitive cultures who survive to the age of 60 years often remain free of them, unlike their "civilised" counterparts. Cardiovascular diseases and cancers, and also hypertension and diabetes, became common in Western society as dietary habits changed over the last 100 years.

Eaton and Konner argue that natural selection has provided us with nutritional adaptability. But we have moved outside the range of fitting foods by the development of agriculture, especially recent agribusiness and food-processing. Ancestors of ours began to consume considerable amounts of meat between 1.8 and 1.6 million years ago, in addition to food from plant sources. Shells and shellfish came later. In periods with stagnant big game hunting, a shift to agriculture reduced the intake of animal protein, with the result that people became shorter and experienced diseases of malnutrition. Nowadays, we in "civilised" regions have adequate amounts of animal protein, but in other respects our diet is inadequate. We suffer from "affluent malnutrition."

By and large, we can reconstruct the diets of our ancestors, and we also know about the diets of existing hunter-gatherers in marginal habitats, which are rather similar. From this we can infer what kind of diet would be appropriate for ourselves. Meat from game would be excellent, but meat from our domestic livestock is less healthy, as it contains far less polyunsaturated fat, particularly omega-3 PUFAs, which have antiatherosclerotic properties. Another significant point is that small cereal grains, which have been staples for "civilised" people since the agricultural revolution, make a surprisingly small contribution to the diets of hunter-gatherers. They eat a wide variety of vegetable foods. Meat and fish, together with vegetables and fruit, form the main constituents of the hunter-gatherer's diet. We have added to this much milk and milk products, and bread and cereals, which represents a highly unnatural situation. Eaton and Konner present many more details, concerning fibre, minerals, and vitamins. They note that accumulating evidence suggests that we would benefit from a change in the direction of the hunter-gatherer diet. Many of their suggestions have been borne out by later research, as put together in the reviews by Simopoulos (1991, 1997, 1999 and 2001a). What follows is a summary of Simopoulos (2001a).

Simopoulos first of all points to the significance of the Seven Countries Study, the first to establish credible data on cardiovascular disease prevalence rates in seven countries (United States, Finland, The Netherlands, Italy, former Yugoslavia, Japan and Greece), the results of which were published more than thirty years ago by Keys (1970). In Greece, the Isle of Crete was the location chosen. The common diet there resembles the traditional diet of Greece before 1960. Earlier studies had already shown that Crete has the lowest death rate in the Mediterranean area, and that cancer and heart disease cause almost three times as many deaths in United States as in Crete. The Seven Countries Study revealed differences among countries in coronary heart disease in the order of 5- to 10-fold. Relations between diet, particularly the fatty acid composition, and heart disease, are clearly in evidence. The results confirm the idea that our diet should be consistent with our evolution.

The investigators doing the Seven Countries Study found that Crete had the lowest rates of cardiovascular disease and cancer. They attributed this to the high olive oil intake and the low saturated fat intake in Crete. Simopoulos presents a more refined analysis. She argues that the traditional diet of Greece resembles the Palaeolithic diet in terms of fibre, antioxidants, saturated fat, monounsaturated fat, and the ratio of omega-6 to omega-3 fatty acids. Western diets deviate from this. They are associated with high rates of cardiovascular disease, diabetes, obesity and cancer.

People in Crete have much fat in their diet. They eat a lot of fish, and large amounts of vegetables, fruits, nuts and legumes. This kind of diet has a high omega-3 content, a low omega-6 to omega-3 ratio, and a rich variety of antioxidants (which are needed alongside omega-3 acids), minerals and vitamins. Purslane is cherished, so that the people take in much LNA (see the previous section).

The Lyon Heart Study, done in the 1990s, confirms that the Crete diet is healthy. The study was set up as a prospective randomised trial in which a modified Crete diet was compared with a diet recommended by the American Heart Association (AHA) over a period of five years. The Crete diet showed a comparative decrease in death rate by 70 per cent, with a clear decline of heart disease and cancer. It was clearly superior to the AHA diet (for comments on the AHA, see also Section 2).

A large literature reviewed by Simopoulos provides a rich variety of additional confirmatory evidence: data from animal experiments, additional epidemiological data, knowledge concerning the mechanisms by which omega-3 PUFAs provide protection, and positive results of clinical trials with these acids. Recent articles keep confirming that omega-3 PUFAs help to prevent heart disease (Christensen and Schmidt, 2001; Harper and Jacobson, 2001; Kristensen *et al.*, 2001; Leaf, 2001; Nordoy *et al.*, 2001; Albert *et al.*, 2002; Bucher *et al.*, 2002; Hu *et al.*, 2002). Likewise for cancer (Albino *et al.*, 2000; Narayanan *et al.*, 2001). In cancer, the omega-3 PUFAs even have beneficial effects in advanced illness characterised by cachexia, a condition of wasting away with pronounced weight loss. Fish oil, which is rich in omega-3 PUFAs, may reverse the weight loss, improve the quality of life, and increase life span (Barber, 2001; Barber *et al.*, 2001). All in all, the evidence that we need omega-3 PUFAs to stay healthy is overwhelming.

Unfortunately, the good news that omega-3 PUFAs may enhance our well-being keeps being overwhelmed by research with a different message. Phillips (2003), in a recent overview in the *New scientist*, reports that researchers are discovering that cholesterol as a cause of clogged arteries is only half the story (she does not recognise it as a myth, as we did; see Section 2). Common opinion is now switching to the view that atherosclerosis is also a matter of inflammation (adhesion of immune cells to the endothelium, the inner lining of blood vessels), so that the immune system has to play a role. This is in keeping with associations between heart disease and many types of infection, which have been noticed for a long time. The industry is developing new drugs that counteract the role of newly discovered pro-inflammatory substances, and results of ongoing research into this possibility are underway. This is presented as good news, but it is only half the story of inflammation. The issue of inflammation is in fact old news that has been kept at the margin of medical research and medical practice. The untold half of the story is about relations between omega-3 PUFAs and inflammation, which calls for diet therapies rather than a new drug wave.

7.5. Conclusions

1. Official nutrient guidelines are often inadequate as a result of biased research influenced by the industry. The "cholesterol myth" of cardiovascular disease is a telling example.

2. During the last century, diets in Western countries have deteriorated. New forms of agriculture and husbandry and new food processing methods cause marked deficiencies of omega-3 polyunsaturated fatty acids (PUFAs) in our food. Omega-3 PUFAs play essential roles in the functioning of cell membranes and they are converted in the body into important hormone-like substances. Thus, they affect numerous physiological functions. This explains the high prevalence of many somatic and psychiatric illnesses in populations where omega-3 shortages are common.

3. Scientific evidence of omega-3 deficiencies has been available since long, but it was disregarded by most medical professionals and health care authorities.

4. Epidemiological studies confirmed the significance of omega-3 PUFAs. Epidemiology has uncovered correlations between diet, the

prevalence of particular diseases, and lifespan. Prospective controlled long-term studies also show that diets which are rich in omega-3 PUFAs have beneficial effects.

5. A great variety of additional evidence further confirms the significance of omega-3 PUFAs. Many diseases are indeed associated with low blood levels of omega-3 PUFAs. Randomised controlled trials (RCTs) demonstrate that treatment with omega-3 PUFAs has preventive and curative effects in many diseases. Furthermore, reconstructions of our evolutionary past indicate that diets rich in omega-3 PUFAs should be natural for us.

Chapter 8

Drugs *Versus* Diets

8.1. Introduction

On December 19 of the year 2000, NOVA, an important news-of-the-day TV program in The Netherlands, presents a fight between pharmaceutical industries over omeprazole (trade name Losec), one of the wonder drugs against gastric ulcers that were introduced a few decades ago.

About 2 per cent of the general population in The Netherlands depends on omeprazole. The drug is an "antacid" belonging to the so-called proton pump inhibitors, which reduce the secretion of acid by cells in the stomach. It is produced by Astra Zeneca, a pharmaceutical company that makes huge profits with omeprazole sales alone, since the drug is expensive. As the expiration date of the omeprazole patent was imminent, other industries were about to take over the market with much cheaper analogues of omeprazole. The financial benefits for health care in The Netherlands would be considerable: Cheaper variants of omeprazole would reduce yearly costs of the medication by approximately US $ 350,000,000. Astra Zeneca attempts to prevent the loss of profits by legal tricks aiming at a new patent that should last until the year 2014. The TV program presents interviews with participants in the ongoing struggle: representatives of industries, and a member of Dutch parliament who had been a General Practitioner (a pivotal profession in Dutch health care). The Member of Parliament is furious about the threat of a financial disaster from Astra Zeneca. He appeals to the body politic to prevent tricks with patents on medications that benefit many persons, as the costs would be outrageous. As we are writing this, a happy end of the story has not materialised: pharmaceutical companies are still fighting over the issue in courts of law. Pending the trials, omeprazole continues to hold a dominant, immensely profitable share of the market.

The story is a telling example of how vested interests affect health care. We applaud that the fight over finance associated with patent rights was raised to public awareness. But the issue of finance detracted from more serious problems. The massive use of omeprazole should have been exposed as the main problem. Some persons may benefit from the drug, but in most cases different, cheaper treatments are advisable (Van der Steen and Ho, 2001b).

We already discussed overmedication with psychotropic drugs in Chapter 6. The case study in the present chapter concentrates on omeprazole and the non-steroid anti-inflammatory drugs (NSAIDs); it is an extension of an analysis in Van der Steen and Ho (2001b). Like omeprazole, NSAIDs have a large share of the Western drug market. They were originally targeted against chronic inflammatory diseases such as rheumatoid arthritis (for a description of this disease, which may be crippling, see Chapter 2.4). Nowadays, NSAIDs are used in large quantities, as they are also prescribed as analgesics against milder complaints such as muscle aches and headaches. Many prescriptions of NSAIDs are indeed unnecessary (Coste *et al.*, 1995; Tamblyn *et al.*, 1997). Sales have increased further since the drugs became available as over-the-counter medications, a few years ago in The Netherlands.

The use of NSAIDs against mild complaints such as muscle aches may be harmless if treatments are limited to short periods. More problematic are high-dose treatments with NSAIDs of autoimmune diseases over long periods. These treatments may not be very effective and they often cause serious gastrointestinal problems, for example ulcers of the stomach and the adjacent part of the gut, the duodenum—gastric ulcers for short. These problems are often treated with antacids, in most cases proton pump inhibitors such as omeprazole. The antacids may also have serious side effects. Thus, we may get caught into vicious circles of runaway medication (for references and comments, see Van der Steen and Ho, 2001b).

NSAIDs are not the only cause of the gastrointestinal problems. Infections with the bacterium *Helicobacter pylori* may play a role in the causation of the ulcers, for example. These infections are generally treated with antacids together with antibiotics for one or two weeks. Spectacular cures may occur, but the treatment does not work in many cases. This invites drug treatment over much longer periods, omeprazole being the most common choice; antibiotics cannot be used over long periods. As omeprazole is also used against milder stomach complaints, sale totals have become impressive. Drugs such as omeprazole may have their uses in the treatment of stomach ulcers. But current prescriptions represent in effect overmedication.

Alternative treatments are available both for the ulcers and for diseases treated with NSAIDs (references are to be found in sections hereafter). In either case, dietary treatments with particular polyunsaturated fatty acids (PUFAs, especially the omega-3 acids eicosapentaenoic acid, EPA, and docosahexaenoic acid, DHA) present in fish oil may help prevent these diseases. Less certain is the feasibility of cures. But, in the case of autoimmune diseases, NSAIDs do not effect cures either; at best they alleviate symptoms. Fatty acid treatments could be a better option as they have few negative side effects, if any. Stomach ulcers are a different matter. Drug treatments may be the best option once the ulcers have developed. But fatty acid treatments may help prevent or even cure milder conditions such as gastritis, and they may also prevent gastritis from leading to ulceration.

It is unfortunate that the emphasis in ongoing research is overwhelmingly on drug treatments since a large share of funding comes from the pharmaceutical industry. Diet treatments with omega-3 PUFAs receive much less attention, even though they should be effective in many chronic diseases and psychiatric disorders. As common diets in Western countries are deficient in these acids, treatment with omega-3 food supplements should be a rational option in many cases (see Chapter 7). We discuss dietary treatments in Section 4. First we provide some details of problems with conventional medications in Sections 2 (NSAIDs) and 3 (antacids and antibiotics). Section 5 comments on views of a philosopher, Thagard, which illustrate the perpetuation of bias in research on stomach ulcers.

8.2. NSAIDs: Vested Interests in Drug Research

The overuse of drugs has become a serious problem. In Section 6.2, we already discussed the case of psychotropic medications, as reviewed by Healy (2002). Healy demonstrated that the pharmaceutical industry, in many cases with the connivance of agencies responsible for regulation, has created overmedication with these drugs in violation of scientific evidence. Science also contributes to this, since funding by the industry causes biased research. Other authors have confirmed that research on drug treatments is biased owing to funding by the industry. An analysis by Fava (2002) suggests that the influence of the industry is indeed more extensive than official sources would admit. Kjaergard and Als-Nielsen (2002) showed that researchers publishing in the British Medical Journal are more likely to be positive towards treatments when their research is funded by for profit organisations, and Bekelman *et al.* (2003) observed the same trend in a more wide-ranging study. Stelfox *et al.* (1998) observed this trend in research on calcium-channel antagonists used to treat cardiovascular disorders, potentially with serious side effects. Djulbegovic *et al.* (2000) report the trend for treatments against multiple myeloma, and Wahlbeck and Adams (1999) for the use of antipsychotic drugs in schizophrenia. Doctors are also influenced by the industry in a more direct way. They are misled by many advertisements of the pharmaceutical industry that refer to clinical trials to back up claims in favour of drugs marketed by them. The claims are often at variance with the publications cited in the adverts (Villanueva *et al.*, 2003).

No reason exists why NSAIDs and omeprazole should be an exception to this general pattern. As to omeprazole, the NOVA story described at the beginning of this chapter is suggestive evidence. We have informally discussed the matter with members of regulatory agencies and persons advising the government. They confirmed that overmedication with omeprazole is unofficially recognised as a major problem. But this sort of information is confidential. We have not uncovered published research on links between the industry and research on omeprazole.

Publications concerning the influence of the industry on the use of NSAIDs do exist. Goetsche (1989) reported that the chances that researchers observe positive effects of NSAIDs are way above average if they are paid by the industry manufacturing the drugs. The most extensive study on NSAIDs has been done by Abraham (1995). He offers a detailed survey spanning decades of NSAID regulation in the United Kingdom and in the United States. The survey demonstrates that research by the pharmaceutical industry on benefits and side effects of NSAIDs has been biased in favour of its own products, and also that authorities responsible for regulation have often taken sides with the industry in violation of their own guidelines. Abraham makes clear that many NSAIDs now on the market should never have been approved for sale; his observation is still valid as we are writing this.

Biased drug regulation invites disasters. Abraham illustrates this by the case of benoxaprofen (trade name Opren in the United Kingdom, Oraflex in the United States). This drug was promoted in the United Kingdom and the United States with the claim that it is an exceptionally effective NSAID in the treatment of arthritic diseases. This claim was based on research conducted by scientists working for the manufacturing industry. However, close examination by other researchers revealed that findings had been selectively emphasised or omitted in support of the assumption that benoxaprofen is clinically more effective than other NSAIDs. The discovery of selectivity did not prevent the regulatory authorities in the two countries from approving the drug for the market. Neither did the inadequate safety assessment conducted on benoxaprofen. The British authorities approved Opren without requiring experimental photosensitivity testing on human subjects and after the completion of only one problematic carcinogenicity test on animals, the tests being clearly indicated. In the United States, Oraflex was approved despite unsatisfactory carcinogenicity tests. In contrast to their permissively approving benoxaprofen, the authorities were reluctant to remove the drug from the market after serious adverse effects had been observed. Patients suffered from photosensitivity reactions and oncholysis (loosening of the nails from the nail beds) and, more seriously, several cases including fatal ones pointed to benoxaprofen-associated toxicity for the kidneys, the gastrointestinal tract and the liver. The growing controversy about the drug's efficacy and safety ultimately forced the manufacturer to withdraw it from the market.

Abraham's analyses show that drugs with known dangerous side effects have been approved for the market without scientific backing. The drug regulation system apparently fails to protect public health, as the pharmaceutical industry's influence on governments and regulatory agencies is overwhelming (Abraham, 2002). For example, since the late 1980s, "European governments ... decided to restructure their drug regulatory authorities in line with the industry's demands" (Abraham *et al.*, 2002: 1165). The industry's influence increased since regulatory agencies have become heavily dependent on industry fees for their survival. As a result, "regulatory bodies have been placed in competition with each other for industry fees, and where there are institutional incentives, not to reject new drugs" (idem: 1165).

Dangerous side effects of NSAIDs are still common. In the remaining part of this section, we present some representative recent findings in brief. The available evidence shows that new varieties of NSAIDs, marketed with the claim that they are safer than classic NSAIDs, are not in fact a safer option.

Patients who use classic NSAIDs in high dosages over prolonged periods may get gastric ulcers (ulcers in the stomach or the duodenum). The drugs may account for more than half of all episodes of ulcer bleeding and perforation; these adverse effects have often resulted in hospitalisation and death (Wolfe, 1996; Griffin, 1998). More recently, Moore (2002) stated that the costs associated with the prevention and treatment of NSAID-induced side effects can more than double the costs of the original therapy: They should be included when costing NSAID interventions. Hawkey (2002) states that NSAIDs account for more reports of drug related toxicity than any other class of drugs. Furthermore, findings by Thomas *et al.* (2002) indicate that medical professionals may overlook gastrointestinal side effects in self-medicating patients using over-the-counter NSAIDs. They conclude that these drugs are dangerous even at low dosages, and therefore suggest that physicians routinely ask patients about all forms of self-treatment.

New classes of NSAIDs, the so-called coxibs, selective cyclo-oxygenase-2 (COX-2) inhibitors, have rapidly gained acceptance in clinical practice. For example, one of these new NSAIDs, celecoxib, became the fastest selling drug in Canada within the first three months of its availability (IMS Health Canada, 1999). The drugs have been widely heralded in medicine, since they allegedly have fewer side effects than classic NSAIDs (see for example Bingham, 2002). The rationale of this assumption concerns the enzymes COX-1 and COX-2. Classic NSAIDs are assumed to inhibit both COX-1, thereby causing the gastrointestinal side effects, and COX-2, thereby causing the desired anti-inflammatory properties. The coxibs are assumed to affect COX-2 only. They are apparently as effective as classic NSAIDs. For example, Lanas (2002) argues that the safety benefits of COX-2 inhibitors given alone appear similar to combined therapy with conventional NSAIDs and gastroprotective agents. He therefore regards COX-2 inhibitors as a first-line therapy in patients requiring long-term pain relief. The use of the new drugs is not restricted to the treatment of inflammatory diseases such as rheumatoid arthritis. According to some authors, they may also diminish chronic pain in cancer and in Alzheimer's disease (Lema, 2002; Staats, 2002).

But the benefits of the coxibs are not unchallenged. The major studies which compared the safety of the main drugs rofecoxib and celecoxib with classic NSAIDs, the Vioxx Gastrointestinal Outcomes Research (VIGOR) trial and the Celecoxib Long-term Arthritis Safety Study (CLASS) trial, have been criticised for biased reporting: While publications on the trials mentioned no difference in the incidence of cardiovascular side effects during the first six months of the trials, the new drugs performed worse when the entire 12-month trial period was accounted for. In correction of these studies, the Food and Drug Administration (FDA) in the United States reported more negative side effects; see the website of the FDA, pages:

- www.fda.gov/ohrms/dockets/ac/01/briefing/3677b1_03_med.pdf
- www.fda.gov/ohrms/dockets/ac01/briefing/3677b1.htm
- www.fda.gov/ohrms/dockets/ac/01/briefing/3677b2_03_med.doc

Jüni *et al.* (2002) comment on the CLASS trial:

> Publishing and distributing overoptimistic short term data using post hoc changes to the protocol, while

> omitting disappointing long term data of two trials, which involved large numbers of volunteers, is misleading. While some of the problems related to CLASS were partially covered in the news sections of … journals, it was not emphasised how flawed the trial actually was, and how inadequate the authors' justifications. Consequently, CLASS may still be relied on by many physicians without reference to these flaws. In our experience most still believe the findings published originally. (Jüni *et al.*, 2002: 1288)

Recent sources confirm that coxibs are not safer than the old NSAIDs. Sica *et al.* (2000) note that existing evidence does not support the claim that coxibs improve on negative side effects of classic NSAIDs affecting the kidney. Peskar *et al.* (2001) add to this that COX-2 inhibitors delay the healing of chronic gastric ulcers in experimental animals. The drugs decrease epithelial cell proliferation, angiogenesis and maturation of the granulation tissue to the same extent as classic NSAIDs. Mengle-Gaw and Schwartz (2002) report that large-scale post-marketing studies have also raised doubts about the safety of coxibs. Kumar *et al.* (2002) describe the case of a patient who died from haemorrhagic pulmonary oedema after taking two doses of the coxib rofecoxib; they also mention heart problems as a known side effect.

The alleged specificity of selective COX-2 inhibitors, coxibs, has also been challenged. The specificity proclaimed by proponents of the coxibs seems a tough call. It is implausible that the actions of any drug could be as specific as those claimed for these drugs. Konstam and Weir (2002) argue that coxibs may have side effects along a biochemical route that differs from the route of classic NSAIDs. The existence of such side effects is still controversial.

As NSAIDs may cause stomach ulcers, their use creates additional problems as drugs against ulcers have side effects of their own. In the next section, we consider these side effects in greater detail. We also consider the aetiology of the ulcers. They may be caused by NSAIDs, but a different route involving infection with the bacterium *Helicobacter pylori* also exists. This route has to be charted in some detail, as views of aetiology motivate particular treatments.

8.3. Gastric Ulcers: Drugs as Magic Bullets?

Gastric ulcers have long been a common protracted illness

worldwide. Recent research has conduced to the view that, barring ulcers caused by NSAIDs, the spiral bacterium *Helicobacter pylori* is the paramount cause of the ulcers. The bacterium lives in the stomach, which for a long time has been regarded as an almost sterile environment in view of its acidity. The presence of spiral bacteria in the stomach had actually been reported over a century ago, but the medical community then considered them as mere contaminants and ignored the reports (Buckley and O'Morain, 1998).

After the spiral bacteria were first cultured from a gastric biopsy specimen in 1982 (see Goodwin, 1994), the Australian physicians Warren and Marshall noticed an association between gastritis and the presence of the bacteria. Gastritis is an inflammation of the mucosa, the inner lining of the stomach. Warren and Marshall's research resulted in their hypothesis that *Helicobacter pylori* infection is the main cause of ulcers, which develop by way of gastritis, and they recommended treatment with antibiotics. The medical community did not accept the hypothesis right away, since the ulcers were generally attributed to excess acidity caused by stress and other factors, to be treated with antacids. General acceptance of the hypothesis was gained with a consensus conference in 1994.

The rate of infections with *Helicobacter pylori* has rapidly increased from the 19th to the 20th century (Lam, 1993; Baron and Sonnenberg, 2001 and 2002). By now, *H. pylori* may be found in up to 50 per cent of the world's population (Lacy and Rosemore, 2001). From a survey on Campogalliano, a town in northern Italy with about 5000 residents, Dominici *et al.* (1999) infer that infection clusters within families belonging to the same population, and that social status may also be a risk factor. According to them, this suggests either a person-to-person transmission or a common source of exposure. As the bacterium is able to withstand immune responses, infections caused by it tend to be chronic (Lohoff *et al.*, 2000).

Most people infected with *H. pylori* never develop symptoms, but some infected persons suffer from gastritis, a mucosal inflammation that may lead to gastric ulcers (Misciagna *et al.*, 2000). The bacterium is also regarded as a risk factor for particular cancers: duodenal ulcer, distal gastric adenocarcinoma and mucosal-associated lymphoid tumour (see for example Farthing *et al.*, 2001). Woodward *et al.* (2001) state that the lowering effect of *H. pylori* infection on vitamin C plasma levels may contribute to gastric cancer and other diseases associated with antioxidant deficiency. In addition to this, the bacterium can infect the skin, the liver and the heart, and it can impair the nutritional status of children and adults (for references, see Lacy and Rosemore, 2001). Some medical professionals recommend for this reason that, whenever infection with *H.*

pylori is diagnosed, it should be treated (Shiotani *et al.*, 2000).

The common therapy against *H. pylori* infections, at least infections associated with ulceration, is nowadays a short-term therapy of one or two weeks with antibiotics and antacids, acid-suppressive drugs. Antibiotics alone are not as effective as this kind of combination therapy. A recent consensus report recommends the use of antacids belonging to the proton-pump inhibitors, particularly omeprazole, along with two or three antibiotics, for a minimum of 7 days (Pilotto and Malfertheiner, 2002; Qasim and O'Morain, 2002). But the therapy should only be used to treat serious conditions (see also Meurer and Bower, 2002). However, eradication rates with such therapies are at best 90 per cent, and resistance against antibiotics is becoming a problem (De Boer and Tytgat, 2000; Trust *et al.*, 2001). To the extent that these therapies do not work, we are back with the antacids which, unlike antibiotics, can be prescribed over long periods *in some cases* without *pronounced* harm. That is why prolonged maintenance therapies with omeprazole are still common (see Section 1).

Omeprazole may cause nausiness, muscle aches, stomachaches, diarrhoea and constipation, and also more serious conditions such as peripheral neuropathy, serious skin damage, renal function failures and acute gout (Cox, 1992; Christensen *et al.*, 1993; Assouad *et al.*, 1994; Jones *et al.*, 1994; Kraus and Flores-Suarez, 1995). Less conspicuous side effects are also a cause for concern. For example, prolonged use of omeprazole may backfire in that gastric acid secretion increases beyond the original level after the cessation of treatment, owing to damaged cells in the inner lining of the stomach, the mucosa. Cessation of the therapy thus becomes a problem (McCloy *et al.*, 1995; Waldum *et al.*, 1996). According to some sources, omeprazole may also foster autoimmune disease (Sivakumar and Dalakas, 1994).

Omeprazole also harms bacteria ensuring a proper functioning of the gut. These so-called commensal bacteria are a natural ecological defence system of the body. As the drug reduces the acidity of the stomach, pathogenic bacteria and other microorganisms with the capability to harm the gut, may become more dangerous. In this situation they more easily pass the stomach unharmed, and then may start harming the patient. Several studies have confirmed that omeprazole does cause infections with bacteria, protozoan parasites and fungi (Reynaert *et al.*, 1995; Sood *et al.*, 1995; Teare *et al.*, 1995; Goenka *et al.*, 1996; Schapira *et al.*, 1996; Garcia Rodriguez and Ruigomez, 1997; Theisen *et al.*, 2000).

Treatments of omeprazole together with antibiotics aggravate this problem. The antibiotics kill off bacteria in the gut. This also promotes infection by pathogens, since commensal bacteria prevent other microorganisms from settling down in the gut. Apart from this, we are saddled with the resistance problem: Antibiotics have caused and continue to cause the rise of resistant pathogens.

NSAIDs as a cause of stomach ulcers make the situation even more complicated. These drugs represent a separate causal route toward ulceration, but the NSAIDs route and the *Helicobacter pylori* route are not entirely unrelated. Some of the patients treated with NSAIDs develop gastric complaints without being infected with *H. pylori*, others do harbour the bacterium. Remarkably, combination therapies of antacids with antibiotics do not improve on antacids alone in the latter category of patients. The antacids help prevent or cure ulcers, but eradication of *H. pylori* does not enhance ulcer healing (Bannwarth *et al.*, 2002; Graham, 2002). Some have reported negative effects upon eradication of the bacterium, for example reflux esophagitis (Ballesteros-Amozurrutia, 2000). Other researchers have even observed positive effects of *H. pylori* (Campbell *et al.*, 2002; Konturek *et al.*, 2002). Positive effects of *H. pylori* may also be found in patients who do not use NSAIDs. Segal (2001) reports that the bacterium is very common in sub-Saharan countries. In these countries, several diseases of the gut including cancers are rare. Segal attributes this to a protective effect of *H. pylori*.

All in all, the evidence does not indicate that the current widespread use of NSAIDs, antacids, and antibiotics is justified. The drugs should be used sparingly, against serious conditions only. Some of the drugs have been heralded as magic bullets. None of them has quite delivered the goods originally envisaged. Omeprazole and other antacids have been characterised as wonder drugs which, after their introduction a few decades ago, improved on existing treatments of gastric ulcers in a spectacular way. The characterisation is deserved, but the drugs did not work in all cases, and they have negative side effects. The discovery of *Helicobacter pylori* as an important cause of the ulcers marked a new phase in the fight against the ulcers. It invited the use of another class of drugs heralded as wonder drugs, antibiotics. The antibiotics appeared to improve on existing treatments with antacids. But as it turned out, the antacids had to remain in force. To some extent, we have solved the ulcer problem, but the use of the drugs is backfiring by way of side effects and antibiotic resistance.

Why should drugs with side effects, serious ones in many cases, be used on such a massive scale? Part of the answer appears to be that the industry has managed to have their use extended from limited domains of application to broad, vaguely delimited domains of mild complaints.

Omeprazole, with or without antibiotics, is an important treatment option in severe cases of ulceration. But we should oppose existing overmedication. In some countries, consensus exists about the necessity to restrict the use of omeprazole. However, actual prescriptions often violate official consensus. Nardino *et al.* (2000) report that 54 per cent of hospitalised patients in a United States hospital received acid-suppressive therapy, with 65 per cent of the prescriptions violating consensus review. Patients were typically discharged with the admonition that they should stay with the medication.

The existing overmedication is deplorable. In many situations, the medications may be inadequate also when no overmedication exists, because better alternatives are available. The next section deals with omega-3 food supplements as potential alternatives.

8.4. Benefits of Fish Oil

Considering the problems with NSAIDs, omeprazole and antibiotics, the search for alternative treatments should be high on the agenda. Most publications on conditions treated with NSAIDs, and ulcers treated with antacids such as omeprazole and antibiotics, suggest that no alternatives are available. But this only reflects the impact of the pharmaceutical industry on research. Alternatives exist, but mainstream research mostly disregards them. Here is an interesting example. Honey has been used during many centuries for the treatment of ulcers, inclusive of gastric ulcers, successfully so (Root-Bernstein and Root-Bernstein, 1997), and it is experiencing a comeback (Dunford *et al.*, 2000; Gharzouli *et al.*, 2001; Natarajan *et al.*, 2001; Alcaraz and Kelly, 2002). Melatonin could also be a promising option (Bandyopadhyay *et al.*, 2001).

Some studies suggest that NSAID treatment had better be replaced by diet treatments (Cleland *et al.*, 1995; Kremer, 1996; Saso, *et al.*, 1999). We focus here on diet therapy with fatty acids. Many patients would presumably benefit from a replacement of drug treatments by treatments with particular polyunsaturated fatty acids (PUFAs), especially the omega-3 acids eicosapentaenoic acid (EPA) and docosahexaenoic acid (DHA). If used as diet supplements, by way of fish oil capsules for example, these PUFAs help to prevent many diseases and disorders, and they may also have curative effects (see Chapters 7 and 10). Unlike pharmaceutical drugs, omega-3 acids do not have undesirable side effects (provided that they are used together with an antioxidant such as vitamin E).

Particular diets containing these PUFAs reduce disease activity in rheumatoid arthritis, a disease which is usually treated with NSAIDs (DeLuca *et al.*, 1995; Rothman *et al.*, 1995; James and Cleland, 1997;

Alexander, 1998; Ariza-Ariza *et al.*, 1998; Mantzioris *et al.*, 2000; Volker *et al.*, 2000). This may be explained in part by known influences of dietary PUFAs on the immune system (Hughes and Pinder, 2000). We review some details for readers who are interested in the theme of fatty acids and immunity:

> PUFAs have the potential to modify immune functions by modulating the production of pro-inflammatory cytokines (Calder, 1997) and other mediators in inflammatory processes, including thromboxanes, prostaglandins, interleukins (James *et al.*, 2000; Kremer, 2000) and pro-inflammatory arachidonate metabolites (Barham *et al.*, 2000). Ergas *et al.* (2002) provide an up-to-date analysis concerning omega-3 fatty acids in immune and autoimmune diseases. They suggest that fish oil with the antioxidant vitamin E helps prevent such diseases by virtue of its anti-inflammatory properties. Fish oil appears to influence T-cells of the immune system (for confirmation, see also Almallah *et al.*, 2000; Grimble, 2001; Terada *et al.*, 2001). The omega-3 acids also have beneficial anti-inflammatory effects by suppressing adhesion of monocytes to human endothelial cells (Mayer *et al.*, 2002; see also Grimm *et al.*, 2002, and Sethi *et al.*, 2002, for more details).
>
> The entire story of fatty acid metabolism and inflammation is complex. In Chapter 7.3 we noted that, according to the received opinion among fatty acid researchers, omega-3 PUFAs and omega-6 PUFAs work in an antagonistic fashion. Omega-3 PUFAs appear to have anti-inflammatory effects, whereas omega-6 PUFAs are pro-inflammatory. The pro-inflammatory effects are not harmful as such. Inflammation is part of the immune defence against infections. But overshoots of inflammation may be harmful. Hence, our bodies need a proper balance of omega-3 and omega-6 PUFAs. As omega-3 acids are in shorter supply in common diets than omega-6 PUFAs, the emphasis in fatty acid treatments has been on food supplements with omega-3 PUFAs. However, the researcher Horrobin, who studies the role of PUFAs in schizophrenia, disagrees with the balance idea (see Chapter 7.3), while agreeing that we

> need omega-3 PUFAs. Studies of rheumatoid arthritis have shown that the truth lies in between these views (for references, see Barham *et al.*, 2000). Several studies have shown that gamma-linolenic acid (GLA), an omega-6 PUFA, actually attenuates symptoms of rheumatoid arthritis by deactivating particular inflammatory processes. But GLA also has some pro-inflammatory side effects (Calder and Zurier, 2001). The side effects can be reduced by EPA. We will not bother you with more details. Suffice it to say that we anyhow need omega-3 PUFAs to keep inflammatory processes from wreaking havoc with our physiological balance.

It is plausible that omega-3 PUFAs should be beneficial also in gastrointestinal disorders. For example, PUFAs in fish oil reduce duodenal ulcers in humans (for references, see Tovey and Hobsley, 1998; Drago *et al.*, 1999). Experiments with rats confirm this effect (Faust *et al.*, 1989; Kresiun *et al.*, 1993; Thompson *et al.*, 1994; Guzel *et al.*, 1995; al-Harbi *et al.*, 1995; Ulak *et al.*, 1995). In keeping with this evidence, several studies indicate that inadequate diets promote gastric and duodenal ulcers (see for example Das, 1998; Elmstahl *et al.*, 1998; Jain *et al.*, 1999). Tovey and Hobsley (1999) state that *Helicobacter pylori* infection may not be the primary cause of duodenal ulceration in cases not associated with NSAIDs, but a secondary complication. Diet may be one of the most important environmental factors contributing to duodenal ulcer (see also Misciagna *et al.*, 2000).

Indirect evidence also suggests that omega-3 PUFAs should be beneficial in gastrointestinal disorders, as effects of *H. pylori* on the immune system are in many ways the opposite of omega-3 effects. Thus, the bacterium may get better chances of becoming pathogenic if the immune system is already impaired by an omega-3 deficiency. Innocenti *et al.* (2002) argue that *H. pylori* does interfere with the immune system. Ernst and Pappo (2001) and Ernst *et al.* (2001) note that the bacterium causes inflammation in this way, as prolonged infection elicits a marked immune response in the stomach. According to Stassi *et al.* (2002), *H. pylori* infection causes gastric pathology via effects on Th1 immune cells. Lohoff *et al.* (2000) present additional details of immune responses to *H. pylori* which suggest that pathological conditions caused by the bacterium have features of autoimmune diseases. The opposite effects of omega-3 PUFAs on the immune system, which should support diet therapies, are seldom noticed in mainstream literature.

The materials presented here suggest that further studies of diet therapies with omega-3 fatty acids are urgently needed. Studies already done are few and far between, but they are promising. It is odd that standard medications, which have side effects and provoke resistance of *H. pylori* against antibiotics, still carry the day.

In the next section, we consider a detailed analysis of the *H. pylori* issue by the philosopher Thagard. His analysis is a sophisticated application of philosophy of science, in a broad, interdisciplinary sense, to discovery and theorising in medicine. Yet, his approach reinforces mainstream views inclusive of the biases we described. An analysis of Thagard's views shows that the drug *versus* diet problem is not exclusively a matter of bias owing to the pharmaceutical industry. The existing bias is strengthened by inertia of research paradigms that keep focussing on restrictive views of aetiology.

8.5. Philosophical Perspectives

Diseases treated with NSAIDs often have elusive or complicated aetiologies. Received opinion has it that the case of stomach ulcers and duodenal ulcers is more perspicuous. Apart from NSAIDs, infection with the bacterium *Helicobacter pylori* is commonly regarded as the most important cause of the ulcers, and treatments are designed to eradicate the bacterium.

For the sake of argument, let us assume that *H. pylori* does causally contribute to the ulcers in some populations (unless NSAIDs are involved), that particular drugs eradicate the bacterium, and that the drugs effect a cure, in most cases without serious side effects. In such a situation, it seems foolish to deny that *H. pylori* is the main culprit and that the drugs represent the best treatment. We defend the view that the denial need not be foolish at all.

Conceivably, the populations studied may have unhealthy habits of food processing and food consumption. Another population—a real or a hypothetical one— with different habits could exhibit different patterns of ulceration and different responses to drugs. Inadequate diets may create conditions for *H. pylori* to behave as a pathogen, and a change towards adequate diets could prevent ulceration and even cure ulcers. If this were indeed true, then inadequate diets would be a cause of *H. pylori* becoming a pathogen, and *H. pylori* would be the next step in the causal chain leading to ulcers. But the inadequate diets would not be detected as a significant cause as long as they represented a constant factor in the populations studied. This example implies that even the most sophisticated, methodologically sound studies of aetiologies and treatments may yield misleading results.

The materials in the foregoing sections show that the example may be realistic. Diets in the West are often deficient in omega-3 PUFAs. The deficiencies contribute to many diseases. The omega-3 PUFAs are a valuable treatment option in many cases. We may reasonably conjecture that this applies to gastric ulcers as well, and some direct and indirect evidence confirms this. Prevention if not cure of the ulcers may thus be achieved by changes in diet. At the very least, the issue calls for more research. Dominant views focussing on *H. pylori* and drug treatments prevent this research from being carried out in a more than marginal way, and funding by drug companies sustains this situation. Ongoing research is thus biased in a self-perpetuating way.

In principle, critical analyses of the situation by impartial investigators, say sociologists of science or philosophers of science could help us recognise this kind of bias. However, it may not be easy for them to turn against mainstream views in medicine. The views of Thagard (1999) illustrate this. His concern is the scientific explanation of disease and his most important example is the explanation of peptic ulcer disease, that is ulcers of the stomach or the duodenum.

Thagard reconstructs the history of the research resulting in the discovery that *Helicobacter pylori* is a significant cause of the ulcers. He explains the ultimate acceptance of the new discovery by integrating social, psychological and methodological analyses. We have here explanations at two levels. At the level of science, a bacterial theory explains ulcers, and at a higher level an integrative meta-theory explains developments in science itself.

Considering meta-theories, Thagard argues that these should conform to the views of scientists themselves: "The main criterion for assessing a model of disease explanation is whether it accounts for the explanatory reasoning of medical researchers and practitioners" (Thagard, 1999: 116). He shows that his theory satisfies this criterion.

The new bacterial theory was at variance with views existing at the time, but these views were problematic:

> In retrospect, there were problems with the accepted view of ulcers. It was not known *why* some people have excess acidity, although conjectures were made about genetic factors and psychological factors such as stress. ... although antacid drugs were usually effective in controlling the symptoms of ulcers, it was well known that the recurrence of ulcers was common: The drugs did not produce a cure. (Thagard, 1999: 58)

The new theory was indeed supported by impressive evidence that the association between bacteria and ulcers represents causation, not mere co-occurrence (idem: 59-64).

Thagard emphasises that the bacterial theory of ulcers must not be construed as a single cause theory. His account of medical explanation takes the form of "causal network instantiation" (idem: 113-115). The causal network for ulcers is a web of interrelated factors with conditions in the stomach (acidity and other factors) at a central node. Miscellaneous factors may cause changes in these conditions, notably: heavy use of NSAIDs as a treatment in arthritis, genetic predisposition, environmental factors (smoking, stress), and *Helicobacter pylori* infection. Increased acidity of the stomach and infection may cause ulceration by different routes, but causal relations also interconnect acidity and infection. As well, causal arrows go from genetic predisposition to increased acidity and from environmental factors to infection. "Given this network, we explain why a given patient has a given disease by instantiating the network, that is, by specifying which factors operate in that patient" (idem: 114).

Thagard's causal network does represent the ulcer theory of mainstream medicine. We regard the network as misleading since the factor of diet is missing. Also missing are details of the immune system, which would explain why diet may be important (see the previous section). Thagard's method of analysis precludes the discovery of the missing factors. We analyse some of his arguments to illustrate this. In one place, Thagard reasons as follows:

> A probabilistic theory of causality would note that the probability of ulcers given the presence of *H. pylori* infection is much higher than the probability of ulcers otherwise. This conclusion is true but irrelevant if the increased probability is accidental or the result of a common cause that encourages both ulcers and bacteria. (Thagard, 1999: 64)

He subsequently argues that additional evidence concerning mechanisms is needed for the inference that *H. pylori* is causally salient in the pathogenesis of ulcers. Such evidence was indeed obtained by researchers. Thus, the new ulcer theory became quite credible.

Thagard does not realise that all the research he considers may have taken place with patients sharing particular features. Such constant features do causally contribute to the results we are getting. Thagard repeatedly disregards this point. For example, with reference to the passage just quoted, he notes that eradication experiments (antibiotics against *H. pylori*) yielded convincing evidence, as alternative causes of the ulcers were excluded: The experiments were done "under circumstances in which no alternative causal factors such as stress, diet, and stomach acidity were varied" (idem: 106). However, we may as well argue that the alternative factors could turn out to be significant causes of the ulcers if they were studied as variables rather than as constants. The alternative factors are irrelevant under conditions as studied in the experiments, and extrapolation of the results to other conditions is formally inadmissible. The advantage of experiments such as those considered by Thagard is that they allow firm conclusions. But we pay a price for this since the control of variables restricts the domain of application of our results.

Had diets been different in the population at large, then we would presumably have arrived at different theories and different treatments. Indeed, given *existing* evidence outside mainstream medicine, it is conceivable that the fuss about *H. pylori* may on balance create a disaster rather than one of the great victories to be attributed to modern medicine.

8.6. Conclusions

1. Pharmaceutical industries and regulatory authorities have been a source of biased information resulting in an excessive use of non-steroid anti-inflammatory drugs (NSAIDs), antacids and antibiotics.

2. Overmedication is enhanced by the neglect of research that could provide health care with better alternatives for drugs. Mainstream medical science and medical practice seem unaware of the beneficial effects of omega-3 PUFAs (polyunsaturated fatty acids) in diseases commonly treated with drugs such as omeprazole, an antacid, and NSAIDs. Unlike omega-3 PUFAs, these drugs have serious side effects. To the extent that the drugs work well, they should be used sparingly, against serious conditions only.

3. NSAIDs may alleviate symptoms of autoimmune disorders such as rheumatoid arthritis, but they may also have serious side effects, for example gastric ulcers (ulcers of the stomach and the duodenum). Coxibs, a new class of NSAIDs that is replacing classic NSAIDs, are being propagated as safer by the industry and by many researchers, but this flies in the face of the evidence.

4. Antacids such as omeprazole (trade name Losec) are often added to NSAIDs to prevent ulceration, but evidence indicates that this is not always appropriate.

5. The bacterium *Helicobacter pylori* is another causal factor in

the aetiology of gastric ulcers, but its importance is overrated. Attempts to eradicate the bacterium with a combination of antacids and antibiotics, now a standard therapy, are not entirely successful. Inadequate diets may be a root cause of the gastric ulcers, with *H. pylori* in a secondary role. Research focussing on the bacterium fails to take this possibility into account.

6. Some direct evidence and much indirect evidence indicates that the immune system is impaired not only in autoimmune diseases but also in gastric ulcer disease. In either case, deficiencies of omega-3 PUFAs in our diet may be an important cause of the symptoms. Treatment with these PUFAs may help prevent the diseases and in some cases have palliative or even curative effects.

7. The existing privilege of drug therapies over diet therapies is supported by a recent philosophical analysis of research on gastric ulcers. It is desirable that resources from the philosophy of science are redirected towards an assessment of existing bias.

Chapter 9

Qualifying Quantitative Methods

9.1. Introduction

A person who is ill may get well after taking a drug. This need not imply that the drug effected the cure. Previous chapters, especially Chapter 4, have shown that it is difficult to distinguish between genuine drug effects and effects due to other factors. In the ideal case, scientific studies of the problem would yield quantitative estimates of drug effects and other effects. We argue that the ideal is utopian owing to fundamental limitations of quantitative science. For continuity, we use examples from the previous chapter. To start with, we recapitulate some of the points made in Chapter 4.

The mere observation that particular patients get well after taking a drug would not tell us much about the drug. Cures may also represent the natural course of a self-limiting condition, and factors unrelated to the drug treatment may also contribute to cures.

Most researchers in medicine regard randomised controlled trials (RCTs) as the best method to assess drug treatments (for details and comments, see Chapter 4). A double-blind set-up is commonly used to distinguish between effects of a treatment and effects of a placebo. With this set-up, doctors and patients are not told which patients are receiving the drug, or the placebo. Even double-blind RCTs need not be reliable. Drugs have side effects, and we get unreliable data if we do not use "active" placebos with similar side effects (see for example Shapiro and Shapiro, 1997a and 1997b).

The most sophisticated RCTs may still yield inconsistent results as clinical trials differ in samples of patients and experimental conditions. We face here a fundamental, irresolvable problem (see for example Chapters 4.2, 5.4 and 6.3). RCTs are done under controlled conditions which can take many forms. Any test result we get is valid only for conditions as existing during the RCT. Change the conditions, and you may get different results. The rigor of RCTs ensures validity for the experimental situation, but it is at the same time a weakness as the outcomes may not apply to real life situations.

These limitations notwithstanding, the consensus among medical professionals appears to be that the RCT is the strongest research tool in causal inference (Ray and Mayan, 2001). In previous chapters, we argued that the extent of the limitations is underestimated. In the present chapter, we strengthen our arguments by pointing at the need of qualitative considerations in the assessment of medical treatments. Representatives of so-called qualitative research would argue that RCTs are meaningless without qualitative appraisals. We consider their views later. First, we present an analysis of our own that relies on analogies between RCTs and risk assessments which have not been noted in literature known to us.

Risk assessments are a familiar phenomenon in modern society. Industries, other private institutions and governments commonly use them in risk management. For example, management decisions concerning the allowable air pollution by an incinerator may be based on estimated thresholds below which pollution is a negligible health risk, or a risk deemed acceptable under prevailing circumstances. Critics of risk-based policies have argued that this will not do, as the assumption that risks can be calculated is dead wrong (Montague, 2000). According to them, risk assessments cannot account for all the factors that significantly affect the environment. Environmental policies based on such assessments have caused cumulative damage of the world's ecosystems. We have to find a new basis for environmental management, since risk assessments cannot help us improve on existing policies. We will make clear that this critique also applies to RCTs.

9.2. Icy Rivers: To Cross or not to Cross

Considering risk assessment, O'Brien (2000) presents a nice fictional story in *Making better environmental decisions: an alternative to risk assessment.*

> Imagine a woman standing by an icy mountain river, intending to cross to the other side. A team of four risk assessors stands behind her, reviewing her situation. The toxicologist says that she ought to wade across the river because it is not toxic, only cold. The cardiologist says she ought to wade across the river because she looks to be young and not already chilled. Her risks of cardiac arrest, therefore, are low. The hydrologist says she ought to wade across the river because he has seen other rivers like this and estimates that this one is not

> more than 4 feet deep and probably has no whirlpools at this location. Finally, the EPA policy specialist says that the woman ought to wade across the river because, compared to global warming, ozone depletion, and loss of species diversity, the risks of her crossing are trivial.
>
> The woman refuses to wade across. "Why?" the risk assessors ask. They show her their calculations, condescendingly explaining to her that her risk of dying while wading across the river is one in 40 million.
>
> Still, the woman refuses to wade across. "Why?" the risk assessors ask again, frustrated by this woman who clearly doesn't understand the nature of risks.
>
> The woman points upstream, and says "Because there is a bridge." (O'Brien, 2000: 3)

O'Brien criticises the common practice of using risk assessments for environmental management. Her fictional story explains her approach. Here is an additional example of our own. Risk-based management is chosen as a method to decide about the construction of a highway. During the planning phase, risk assessors are asked to estimate negative effects of the planned highway on humans and other organisms such as birds and butterflies. The point would be to assess the so-called "assimilative capacity" of these creatures, and of more inclusive wholes such as ecosystems. The assessors would calculate how much damage could be absorbed by the environment without irreversible harm. Decision makers would then impose limits on the damage by requiring that the highway will not overtax assimilative capacities. Or they would accept more damage if it is offset by benefits for humans who will use the highway.

O'Brien argues that such risk-based approaches do not allow of well-founded environmental decision-making, because they are too restrictive. Mere risk assessments are problematic since they cannot cover all options which are potentially available. A decision about the highway would be irresponsible, for example, if the option of making it superfluous by different infrastructural provisions were disregarded. O'Brien nicely makes her point with the analogy of the woman who is supposed to face a choice between wading across an icy river or staying where she is and missing her destination. Risk assessors in the story consider the pros and cons of wading across the river. The dilemma is serious: By crossing the woman might even drown. The woman, however, does not in fact experience this dilemma, because she knows about a different option.

O'Brien (2000: 7) argues that "risk assessments rarely involve serious consideration of viable alternatives." In line with her story of the woman by the river, she pleads for a different approach called alternatives assessment, which envisages viable options disregarded in risk assessments.

> By assessing the risks of hazardous activities and concluding that some level of the activity poses no or insignificant risks of damage, the risk-assessment process generally attempts to obviate consideration of serious alternatives to those activities ... . (O'Brien, 2000: 13)

The term "alternatives" in this passage may cause confusion. In risk assessments, we do envisage alternatives, as we have to decide, for example, either to construct a highway or not to construct it. Alternatives in this sense are not what O'Brien has in mind. Her alternatives are options outside the scope of risk assessments.

In some situations, risk assessments may be appropriate. But O'Brien's analysis uncovers serious limitations. In many situations, factors outside the context considered would expose risk assessment as a risky affair. When we can cross an icy river by a bridge, there is no point in aiming at cold feet.

9.3. Crooked Chairs and RCTs

O'Brien's analysis demonstrates that risk assessments are dangerously narrow. They may fail to accommodate significant factors outside the contexts chosen to make risk estimates feasible. Hence, environmental policies must not be based on risk-based environmental management alone. For similar reasons, the assessment of medical treatments must not be based on RCTs alone.

RCTs are generally heralded as the gold standard in the evaluation of medical treatments. On the analogy of O'Brien's story concerning risk assessments, we present an autobiographical story of one of us (WJS), which entails that the gold of RCTs may not be pure. The story is about the treatment of backache, which is often a difficult problem for medical professionals.

> I once experienced a nasty backache over a long period. As the complaints persisted, I consulted many persons who might be of help, a general

> practitioner and a specialist in orthopaedics among them. The medics, observing no pathology, suggested that I was to have physiotherapy, and also that I needed different shoes to compensate for slight anatomical abnormalities of my feet that might put the wrong kind of pressure on my spine. I did have physiotherapy, and a shoemaker adapted my shoes to my feet with arch supports. Unfortunately, nothing helped.
>
> With this difficult kind of complaint, analgesics are often used to alleviate the symptoms (see Chapter 8). So it seems reasonable in this case, where effective treatments are difficult to find, to use drugs that may alleviate the pain. But I did not wish to take drugs that would merely suppress symptoms. I wanted to discover a cause of the backache, and I was successful in the end. A crooked chair in my university office turned out to be the culprit, the seat being out of alignment with the horizontal plane. For a long time, I had been forcing my spine into a torsion, with pain to warn me that something must be done. When I finally got the message, I replaced the chair, and the backache disappeared.

The story has a happy ending. I eventually identified the chair as the most important cause of the backache, after a thorough examination of my situation at home and at my work. This resulted in an effective chair "treatment."

Analgesics could have alleviated my pain, but with the benefit of hindsight I know that drugs would have been the wrong treatment. Instead, the crooked chair had to be replaced. The professionals did not find out about it. That is not surprising. Crooked chairs are not qualified to enter aetiologies in medical thinking. Yet, the chair had been the most important aetiological factor, and replacing it had been the best "treatment."

This treatment does not qualify for inclusion in an RCT. If it did, then any old factor that affected somebody's health would have to qualify as well. That would create an unmanageable mess. The rigor of RCTs helps us steer away from the mess, but also from potentially valuable treatments. That is why RCTs have limitations like those of risk assessments.

The chair treatment also demonstrates that strong evidence may reside in unexpected quarters. The evidence in the example is strong. The crooked chair did cause the backache. For one thing, replacing it effected a cure, whereas other treatments had not worked. Furthermore, the complaints and the cure are explained by well-confirmed elementary physics and biology. You cannot maintain a good posture on a deviant seat. If your posture is inadequate for a long time, the chances are that your body will protest with pain. It is as simple as that. The chair treatment is not to be honoured by inclusion in RCTs. Indeed, no need exists for it to be so honoured. It already has enough evidence in its favour. This is another reason why the idea that RCTs are a gold standard is suspect. The chair treatment is a single case study. Yet it has more evidential force than many RCTs (see also Chapter 3.2, which presents a single case study of schizophrenia with the same message).

For contrast, consider a hypothetical RCT with a non-steroid anti-inflammatory drug (NSAID), for example ibuprofen, for the treatment of pain. The results of the RCT are encouraging: The data show that the drug alleviates pain symptoms, whereas side effects are relatively mild. Additional RCTs indicate that the drug is effective in comparison with other drugs. Would this imply that the drug is always the best treatment for patients with the pain symptoms? The answer is no: However convincing the test results may be, we cannot rule out that some patients had better replace their crooked office chairs or change particular aspects of their life styles.

It is true that many patients benefit from drugs, and that their complaints may not be alleviated by simply replacing crooked office chairs. But the possibility remains that we may reduce the number of patients depending on NSAIDs considerably by treatment options disregarded in our RCTs. Like risk assessments, RCTs are formally valid only in particular contexts, and the study of factors outside these contexts may make them irrelevant.

Medical professionals cannot account for office chairs and all sorts of other factors outside their field. They would rightly argue that such factors are to be studied by professionals from other disciplines such as psychology, sociology, economics and politics. In ideal situations, which may be hard to realise, they would join efforts with all these professionals to arrive at integrative diagnoses and treatments.

To strengthen our case, we consider one additional hypothetical example. As argued in Chapters 7 and 8, dietary deficiencies, especially deficiencies of particular omega-3 fatty acids, are pervasive in "civilised" countries. Hence, the chances are that, in these countries, patients in RCTs suffer from these deficiencies. If we perform RCTs with such patients to find out whether some NSAID alleviates their pain symptoms, the outcomes are only valid for persons with the deficiencies. Suppose that we get encouraging results: The data show that the drug investigated alleviates the pain symptoms, and side effects are relatively mild. Also, the drug is shown to outperform other drugs. In this situation, changes in diet could drastically alter the outcomes of drug treatments. As well, treatment of the deficiencies with food supplements may give better results than the drug treatments. Published studies do indicate that many patients using NSAIDs would be better off if they replaced NSAIDs by fish oil, which contains omega-3 fatty acids that are often in short supply in diets; rheumatoid arthritis is presumably an example (see Chapters 7 and 8; in Chapter 8.5 we made the same formal point in a case study of gastric ulcers).

Crooked chairs obviously do not belong to the furniture of medicine. But the study of diet should belong to the core of medicine, as it represents plain biology in the form of ecology. Unfortunately, ecological factors are often disregarded by medical professionals (Chivian *et al.*, 1993; Garrett, 1994; see also Chapters 7 and 8). This is a cause for concern, as we may be overlooking important causes of disease, and effective treatments.

The mainstream, quantitative approach in biomedicine that uses RCTs has also been criticised by representatives of qualitative research, who promote qualitative approaches on the ground that the deliveries of quantitative research are inadequate in clinical situations. In the next section, we explain the nature of qualitative research, and the criticism of RCTs associated with it.

9.4. Quantitative *Versus* Qualitative Research

RCTs represent a quantitative approach in medical research. Qualitative researchers obtain medical data with other methods, for example unstructured interviews and the use of question forms. These methods derive from sources in medicine, psychology, sociology, anthropology and nursing. In *The nature of qualitative evidence*, Morse *et al.* (2001a) examine the nature of qualitative research.

Most scientists would grant that we need both quantitative and qualitative approaches. But, with the rise of so-called Evidence-Based Medicine in the 1990s, qualitative research has been put on a sidetrack by the medical profession (see Chapters 4 and 6.3 for critical comments; Chapter 6.3 also deals with the history of this development). Advocates of Evidence-Based Medicine characterise their approach as the conscientious, explicit and judicious use of best evidence in making health care decisions (Sackett *et al.*, 1996). They recognise a hierarchy of evidence based on the rigour of study design (Upshur, 2001). Evidence from RCTs is at the top of the hierarchy. As Madjar and Walton (2001) put it:

> Thus, while the importance of other forms of knowledge and evidence is acknowledged, the emphasis is predominantly on research evidence derived from RCTs and on systematic reviews and meta-analyses of the findings of experimental research. The standards for evaluation of evidence adopted by the Cochrane Collaboration, the United States Preventive Services Task Force, and the Australian National Health and Medical Research Council clearly privilege some forms of evidence over others. (Madjar and Walton, 2001: 33)

The hierarchy of evidence is endorsed by the Cochrane Collaboration, the international support structure of Evidence-Based Medicine. The Cochrane Criteria have statistically reliable RCTs at the top. At the next lower level of evidential force we find RCTs with uncertain results. Below this level we have non-randomised concurrent cohort comparisons, then non-randomised comparisons with an evidentially weaker format. Case studies and descriptive studies are at the lowest level. Most Cochrane reviews are based on RCTs. By now, the Cochrane Criteria are commonly applied to the evaluation of research proposals and the allocation of money by medical funding agencies. For many of the funding agencies, research is adequate only if it has a large sampled, randomised, experimental research design (Morse *et al.*, 2001b).

Representatives of qualitative research do not question the pertinence of the Cochrane Criteria for the assessment of treatments. They do argue that RCTs and other quantitative research methods have serious limits and limitations which did not receive the attention they deserve. For one thing, RCTs and allied research methods cannot deal with the complicated nature of medical practice. Representativeness thus becomes a problem. RCTs are generally done with restricted patient groups:

> Older adults, those who are too ill or unable to communicate in the language of the researchers, people with cognitive or communication impairments, and many others are frequently excluded from RCTs. ... Extreme scores may be disregarded or excluded from calculations with aggregate data relating to the average patient—a statistical construction bearing limited resemblance to the actual persons encountered in clinical practice. (Madjar and Walton, 2001: 36)

Thus, quantitative work faces insurmountable problems in extrapolations from patient samples to the population at large.

This situation is inevitable for practical reasons, as "the aim of the researcher designing RCTs is to remove individual and contextual differences in order to provide answers to carefully formulated research questions and produce generalizable findings" (idem: 39). But doctors have to deal with individuals and contexts, as all kinds of factors affect patients' diseases and treatment effects (see Chapter 2 and 5). "Dealing with individual patients requires scientific evidence and a great deal more" (idem: 37). The researchers question the hierarchy of evidence advocated in Evidence-Based Medicine. As Upshur (2001) puts it:

> ... evidence in health care is neither exclusively abstract, mathematical, and general nor narrative and particular, but is a mediation and interaction of both types of knowledge. The issues become problematic only when one wishes a monolithic conception of evidence, that is, a single criterion to reliably distinguish truth from falsehood. (Upshur, 2001: 11)

Fuller (2002), professor of sociology, criticises the overwhelming use of Evidence-Based Medicine in Britain for similar reasons. He foresees deteriorations in health care where policy makers promoting Evidence-Based Medicine get their way:

> Firstly, evidence-based medicine deprofessionalises biomedical researchers by stripping away the distinctive assumptions and limitations of their findings. The same applies to clinicians, who are discouraged from relying on their own practical experience. Finally, and paradoxically, it disempowers ordinary citizens because it provides them with a false sense of security about medical findings without the necessary background to make more discriminating judgements.
>
> It should therefore come as no surprise that there is little evidence that evidence-based medicine has actually improved healthcare. (Fuller, 2002: 47)

By solely depending on the Cochrane Criteria of evidence, medical professionals undermine their work as clinical knowledge is overrun by the assumption that quantitative methods alone can determine the best treatment option for patients.

According to Fuller (2002), it is not hard to understand why Evidence-Based Medicine is so actively promoted. The identification of biomedical research with success rates provides free publicity for the pharmaceutical industries supplying allegedly successful treatments. Evidence-Based Medicine also enables politicians to bend situations to their will:

> Their appeal to statistics can claim scientific authority without bothering with potentially awkward scientists. At the same time, they can then blame those very scientists if policies go awry. Of course science should inform policy, but as flesh-and-blood scientists, and certainly not as pre-packaged black boxes of facts. (Fuller, 2002: 47)

In psychiatry, Evidence-Based Medicine with its emphasis on quantitative approaches, has also become a problem. Healy (2002), whose views we have discussed at length in Chapter 6.3, shows that psychiatry became a cultural disaster as qualitative methods gave way to quantitative methods:

> Whereas the nineteenth-century mapping of new domains was largely qualitative (descriptive), twentieth-century mapping was quantitative. The quantitative mapping of IQ and other psychological functions powerfully introduced the notion of a norm and of deviations from that norm into considerations of behavior, giving rise in the process to new concepts, such as that of personality disorder. Whereas qualitative approaches had targeted a limited number of patients, statistical approaches to psychological tests led scientists to claim that they could extrapolate from small samples to the population at large. All of a sudden large groups of people found out that they were abnormal. (Healy, 2002: 349)

As the quantitative mapping filtered through to the institutional level, little room was left for clinical judgments: "the behavior of clinicians is now progressively less likely to be based on knowledge derived from direct clinical encounters" (idem: 350).

The most fundamental limitations of quantitative methods ensue from the necessity of making methodological choices. As the rigor of RCTs increases, their clinical relevance decreases. Hence, we have to make a choice. Either we opt for rigor and sacrifice clinical relevance, or we opt for clinical relevance and sacrifice rigor. As we have to choose between methods, the methods themselves cannot provide us with criteria of choice. We need external criteria, from ethics for example. Hence, qualitative considerations play a crucial role even in the use of RCTs.

Methodological choices cannot be avoided either in statistical analyses. We illustrate this with the problem of false positives (statistical Type I errors) and false negatives (statistical Type II errors). For research to be acceptable, the probabilities of errors of either kind have to be low. The trouble is that a decrease in one type of error logically entails an increase in the other type of error (with a given sample size and effect size). Thus, we need criteria from outside statistics to decide about the set-up of our investigations. We come here across another point of similarity between risk assessments and RCTs. Considering risk assessment, Ashford (1999) characterises the problem as follows:

> Value judgments clearly attend decisions whether to lean toward tolerating Type I or Type II errors with regard to both risk and technology choices. This is because the cost of being wrong in one instance may be vastly different from the cost of being wrong in another. For example, banning a chemical essential to a beneficial activity such as the use of radionuclides in medicine has potentially more drastic consequences than banning a nonessential chemical for which there is close, cost-comparable substitute. It may be perfectly appropriate to rely on "most likely" estimates of risk in the first case and on "worst-case" analysis in the second. (Ashford, 1999: 203)

The choices to be made in RCTs are a matter of ethics. Patients and the pharmaceutical industry have different interests with respect to different types of statistical error. In the interest of patients, Type I errors of falsely attributing positive effects to drugs should be minimised. But the industry would rather benefit from low levels of Type II errors of falsely attributing no effects to drugs.

Remarkably, this problem is seldom mentioned in publications on RCTs. Neither is it a theme in medical ethics. Researchers in medical ethics have useful things to say about themes such as abortion and euthanasia. They should also be concerned with our manners of making sums.

9.5. Conclusions

1. Evidence-Based Medicine, with its preference for randomised controlled trials (RCTs) is commonly regarded as the best approach of research on medical treatments. But RCTs have many limitations.

2. RCTs and risk assessments have much in common. Like risk assessments, RCTs necessarily focus on a restricted set of factors. Factors disregarded may make analyses irrelevant once they are taken into account. This does not imply that RCTs are worthless. They are not. But we have to supplement them with qualitative approaches.

3. It is impossible for scientific methods and theories to meet all methodological requirements that are reasonable in themselves. Hence we face a trade-off problem that is seldom made explicit in ongoing research. We need “external” criteria to prioritise requirements so that they fit with the context of interest. This is an important reason why the value of RCTs is limited.

4. In some situations, factors disregarded in RCTs are known to influence the condition for which a treatment is sought. Deficiencies of omega-3 fatty acids in our diet are known to influence many chronic diseases, for example autoimmune diseases such as rheumatoid arthritis. Most RCTs merely assess drug treatments for these diseases. This may yield misleading results, because diet treatments are not considered as an option.

5. Other factors outside the scope of RCTs cannot within reason be regarded as belonging to medicine, however significant their effects on health may be. If you have a chronic backache caused by a crooked chair in your office, attending doctors presumably will not find out about it. Crooked chairs are not their business. Unfortunately, this kind of situation implies that many patients do not get the right diagnosis and the right treatment, since numerous causes of disease are outside medicine’s field of vision. This is an unacceptable situation. We could change it by redrawing boundaries of medicine, or else by forging more extensive links between medicine and other disciplines.

Chapter 10

Thought for Food in Psychiatry

10.1. Introduction

Drugs or diets? That question has been before us in several chapters. Materials in Chapter 6 indicate that overmedication is common in psychiatry. The general overview of dietary deficiencies and diet treatments in Chapter 7 shows that treatments with omega-3 polyunsaturated fatty acids (PUFAs) are beneficial in many diseases, inclusive of psychiatric disorders. Chapter 8 provides more detailed case studies showing that drug treatments may have to be replaced by diet treatments, in particular in the case of autoimmune diseases and gastrointestinal disorders.

The issue of drugs *versus* diet is a cause for concern in psychiatry since overuse of drugs has become pervasive, whereas potential benefits of diet treatments are vastly underrated. Psychotropic drugs may benefit some patients, but they often have serious side effects (for examples, see Chapters 4.3 and 6.3). "Antipsychotics," for example, may cause irreversible brain damage when used over long periods of time. In many cases, diet treatments should be a more promising option. If patients have shortages of particular essential fatty acids in their diet, then treatment with these acids may benefit them without harmful side effects. Therefore, diet therapies rather than drug therapies deserve the benefit of doubt when either option is available to the practitioner. Diet therapies should also be privileged over drug therapies as subjects of research. Unfortunately, the opposite situation now exists owing to vested interests of the industry.

We review in this chapter the role of omega-3 PUFAs in mental illnesses (for general information on these acids, see Chapter 7 and Section 4 of the present chapter). For contrast we comment on prevailing drug treatments in Section 2, and on theories associated with these treatments in Section 3. The remaining sections provide evidence and general arguments in favour of treatments with omega-3 PUFAs.

We discuss randomised controlled trials (RCTs) as a source of evidence in favour of these treatments. This has to be justified. We have criticised RCTs in Chapters 4, 6, 8 and 9, and now we rely on them to make our own case. That looks like a serious inconsistency. We do not plead guilty, though. RCTs are indeed problematic when they are the sole source of evidence; they have to be supplemented with different varieties of evidence. Evidence supplementing RCTs in support of drug treatments is weak—or so we will argue. Furthermore, tests of drug treatments by RCTs are often suspect since drug companies provide funds. Diet treatments do have additional evidence in their favour, and they are less easily biased by funding.

10.2. Drugs in Psychiatry: Benefit or Burden?

In Chapter 4.3, we surveyed problems with psychotropic drugs. These drugs may have their uses in severe psychiatric disorders, but the signs are that the present use is excessive. They are often marketed on the basis of methodologically problematic RCTs. Some drugs may not have beneficial effects at all, and serious side effects have been noticed (for sources, see Chapter 4.3). The influence of the pharmaceutical industry on research enhances overmedication; we reviewed relations between the industry and research in Chapter 6.3, using a book by Healy (2002) on the history of psychopharmacology. Healy convincingly shows that, over several decades, pharmaceutical companies have managed to sell their products in increasing quantities without proper evidence. His evidence indicates that problems of daily life are often treated with harmful chemicals. Healy's view is confirmed by other recent studies.

Publication bias reinforces this trend. Several studies demonstrated that associations exist between RCT outcomes and funding (for references, see Chapter 8.2). A drug has the best chance of being recommended when the author doing the recommending is paid by the industry marketing it. This kind of publication bias is enhanced by selectivity on the part of the industry. Positive outcomes of trials are likely to be published whereas studies without such outcomes mostly face oblivion. But the industry has to account for them in marketing proposals. In the United States, the Food and Drug Administration (FDA) approves of the marketing of a drug on the basis of two studies with positive outcomes, even if several other studies failed to establish any effect of the drug. This is one of the factors that has boosted the use of antidepressants to unprecedented heights (Kirsch *et al.*, 2002).

The overuse of the drugs fostered by the industry is part of a cultural pattern of medicalisation. Official figures indicate that the prevalence of mental illnesses has become unbelievably high. In England, the annual number of antidepressant prescriptions has more than doubled over the past seven years (Double, 2002). A similar development has occurred in the United States (Kirsch *et al.*, 2002). This development took place while doubts concerning the effects of these drugs are increasingly justified, since studies of treatment effects are flawed (Even *et al.*, 2000; Moncrieff, 2001; Kirsch *et al.*, 2002, and responses following their article; see also Chapter 4). Furthermore, meta-analysis of more adequate studies indicates that the outcomes of trials represent placebo effects (Kirsch and Sapirstein, 1999). Positive outcomes have been observed in some studies, but the effects are typically minor (Kirsch *et al.*, 2002).

Double (2002) notes that the number of consultant psychiatrists has more than doubled over the past 22 years. The proportion of men and women with a neurotic disorder in a given week was 12.3 per cent and 19.5 per cent respectively according to the largest epidemiological study of psychiatric disorders in the United Kingdom. The diagnosis of attention-deficit / hyperactivity disorder with attendant drug prescription in children has recently increased dramatically, in the United States, and now also in the United Kingdom. Paroxetine, originally marketed as an antidepressant, the drug with the greatest net ingredient cost to the National Health Servive (NHS) in England in 2000, is now approved in the United States for use in multiple disorders: depression, generalised anxiety disorder, social anxiety disorder, panic disorder, obsessive-compulsive disorder and post-traumatic stress disorder. Drugs such as this one have indeed been promoted and used as lifestyle drugs.

The phenomenon of multi-purpose drugs is unfortunately gaining momentum (see, for example, Kelleher *et al.*, 2002, who appear to accept it as a matter of course). We do hope that authorities responsible for drug regulation will become aware that such drugs may well prove to cause multi-antipurpose side effects.

Double (2002) sees in all this a negative trend of medicalisation that transforms ordinary problems of living into illnesses to be treated with drugs. We are afraid that, overall, the trend is that persons who during their lives never get a psychiatric diagnosis and a drug going with it, may soon constitute an odd minority.

The sources reviewed here add up to the following overall picture. We are plagued nowadays by overmedication and overdiagnosis of psychiatric disorders. This should not detract from appropriate forms of medications, which also exist. The account that follows is based on personal experience of one of us (FJK), who worked in psychiatry as a medical doctor during the past six years in a clinical setting.

In my (FJK's) experience, some 25 per cent of patients who have a clinically serious psychosis do improve on antipsychotics. Also, some patients with a clinically serious depression appear to benefit from antidepressives. I have to add that such observations do not prove in the way of Evidence-Based Medicine that the drugs were being effective. So much for the good news. The bad news is that many patients did not respond at all, not even when all sorts of medication were tried out in succession. Some of those who did not respond to the first drug they received, would improve somewhat on the second or third drug tried out, but the majority of the patients would stay seriously ill. Aged patients with hallucinations constitute the most difficult category. Serious forms of hallucination seldom improve upon medication. With adolescents who have a serious psychosis, we face the same problem, albeit to a slightly lesser extent. Some of the treatment-resistant patients showed a positive response to electroconvulsive therapy. This old treatment may deserve to be reinstated.

The results obtained with psychotropic medications remain meagre. In my experience, some of the patients with serious symptoms who do not respond to medication improve with psychotherapy. This confirms views of researchers in psychotherapy research (see Chapter 4.3). Fatty acid therapies may even be more promising. I would plead for more research into these therapies.

10.3. From Brains to Drugs and Back Again

Theoretical reasoning in biological psychiatry about brain mechanisms in psychiatric disorders on the one hand, and mechanisms of drug action on the other hand, reveal how existing paradigms are self-perpetuatingly kept alive. The article by Binder *et al.* (2001) on schizophrenia is a representative example. They argue that it is clear by now that the mechanisms responsible for the disorder operate by interacting neurotransmitter systems rather than a single system. We agree: Systems in our body *never* operate in isolation. The authors then suggest that a particular substance, neurotensin, is implicated in schizophrenia, because it modulates all the neurotransmitters systems involved in this disorder. They indicate that neurotensin and antipsychotics have similar effects, and that neurotensin may be regarded as an endogenous antipsychotic.

If this line of reasoning were carried through to its natural conclusion, we would have to conclude that our bodies produce numerous substances that mimic processes like the ones set in motion by psychotropic drugs. Something is terribly wrong here. First, schizophrenia is a non-entity, as argued in Chapter 6. Second, patients who belong to the heterogeneous group of "schizophrenics" are *necessarily* different *in many ways* from other persons. The same goes for persons with the flu *versus* other persons, for example. A selective focus on particular differences does not tell us much in the absence of a theory that justifies the focus. No such theory is here on offer. Third, the reasoning of the authors could as well be applied to any other substance in the biochemical network they are considering, precisely because all the substances are interacting. Why then, single out neurotensin? The authors presumably did this because nobody happened to consider this particular substance beforehand. Had the order of consideration been different, then we would have had a different substance at centre stage. Fourth, whatever associations we find between schizophrenia and biochemical characteristics, we are not allowed to regard the characteristics as pathological unless we have independent arguments for biological pathology (see Chapter 6.1). Such arguments are missing in this case. As we argue in Section 4, theories concerning fatty acids do have credentials in the form of independent arguments.

A simple search of the literature easily uncovers many "theories" of schizophrenia with a similar mode of reasoning and a similar message. We estimate that at least a hundred new theories must have seen the light during the last few years. Here is another example. Konradi and Heckers (2001) have observed particular changes in the brain induced by drugs commonly used in schizophrenia. They are interested in changes in synapses, little organs with clefts separating interconnected nerve cells, which play an important role in the transmission of signals. Drugs appear to influence synapses, so now we have schizophrenia as a disorder of synaptic disorganisation on our hands.

This theory, like many other theories, is grounded on the idea that drugs have particular effects. Let us make clear by an analogy how the reasoning goes. You have a sore throat and a high fever. After having taken antibiotics, you get well again. During the cure and a period of a few days afterwards, you have bowel complaints that necessitate frequent visits to the washroom. (You should have used B vitamins with the antibiotics to prevent this.) What are we to conclude from this? The drug induced bowel complaints. Hence, to understand sore throats, we must know more about mechanisms of bowel action.

Something is obviously wrong with this line of reasoning. But then arguments with the same structure about brain mechanisms responsible for schizophrenia must be wrong by the same token as long as additional, independent evidence is not forthcoming. Researchers in biological psychiatry keep arguing in this way, so far without a clue of pathology *biologically* defined.

However, mental illnesses do appear to have significant

biological aspects. We are going to argue that fatty acid biochemistry provides clues that have been disregarded in mainstream psychiatry.

10.4. Fatty Acids Revisited

Mental illnesses are real in the sense that some persons suffer from severe impairments of cognitive functioning and behaviour. But the overall category of persons thought to have a disorder has been extended to excess. This hampers the recognition of the real thing. In addition to this, problematic classifications hamper the identification of particular forms of mental illness (see Chapter 6).

Psychiatry is not the only discipline responsible for the problems with classification. As Uttal (2001) convincingly argues, psychologists have never been able to devise stable categories for mental phenomena. This awkward situation necessarily carries over to classification of disorders that psychiatrists care to devise.

On top of this, biological variability among human beings, and variability in their antecedent and current circumstances, should preclude a classification of disorders into types with fixed characteristics. Unavoidable variability in the set-up of experiments and other studies on mental illnesses further aggravates this problem. The results obtained are more context-dependent than many researchers would have it.

We assume that mental illness, the real thing, is often accompanied with biological pathology if it is severe. This is not to say that biological factors are necessarily the most significant causes of severe mental illness. Biological pathology may also arise from psychosocial stress. Nor would we assume that mental illness should *always* have biological abnormalities going with it.

As indicated in the previous section, the set-up of much research precludes the discovery of biological abnormalities. Biological psychiatry keeps flooding us with new details concerning the biochemistry of brains in patients that supposedly explain why they are ill. We are missing a serious, coherent theory that moves beyond mere brain biochemistry. The development of an integrative theory with diet in a crucial role is a promising option. In outline, elements for an integrative theory are already available, since long in some cases. In Chapter 7.5, we provided a list of such elements which applies to many diseases. We reproduce it here as it fits with the case of psychiatry in many respects.

- Epidemiological studies reveal correlations between diet, the prevalence of particular diseases, and lifespan. They suggest that shortages of (particular) omega-3 PUFAs impair our health.

- The average diet in the "civilised" countries lacks adequate quantities of omega-3 PUFAs.

- Many diseases are associated with low blood levels of omega-3 PUFAs.

- Prospective controlled long-term studies show that diets which are rich in omega-3 PUFAs have many beneficial effects.

- Randomised controlled trials (RCTs) demonstrate that treatment with omega-3 PUFAs has preventive and curative effects in many diseases.

- Omega-3 PUFAs play essential roles in the functioning of cell membranes and they are converted in the body into important hormone-like substances. Thus, they affect numerous physiological functions.

As to the last point, the immune system deserves special scrutiny, as omega-3 PUFAs influence the balance of pro-inflammatory and anti-inflammatory processes. This tallies with recent research into the role of the immune system in psychiatric disorders. The role of this system may help us come full circle in theorising about psychiatric disorders: Omega-3 deficiencies contribute to psychiatric disorders. Omega-3 deficiencies impair the immune system. The immune system is impaired in psychiatric disorders. It all fits. We are putting it simplistically, but the general idea appears to be sound, the more so as it applies to many more diseases and disorders (Chapter 5.6: migraine; Chapter 7.3 and 7.4: miscellaneous disorders; Chapter 8.4: autoimmune diseases and gastric ulcers). The role of the immune system in many diseases has presumably been undervalued. In part, that is because psychoneuroendocrinoimmunology (PNEI, see Chapter 4.5) is a young discipline. We have been educated into thinking that the nervous system, the hormone system and the immune system are distinct albeit interconnected functional compartments in our bodies. That is not so. The three systems are in fact one system, which interacts with psychological factors in many ways. We emphasise here the aspect of the immune system as it has received relatively little attention in psychiatry.

We list a sample of recent articles which do indicate that immunity is important in psychiatric disorders (for sources concerning omega-3 PUFAs in relation to immunity, see Chapter 7.3; Section 6 surveys evidence of links between omega-3 PUFAs and the disorders). The assumption that the immune system is involved in the disorders is not really new. In particular, the possible role of altered immunity owing to prenatal infection in schizophrenia has been proposed decades ago (Schwarz and Muller *et al.*, 2001). But this proposal has always been controversial. Ongoing research is now yielding more substantial evidence. Considering schizophrenia, Schwarz and Muller *et al.* (2001) suggest that we revive the old infection hypothesis of schizophrenia for a particular subgroup of patients.

Zhang *et al.* (2002) found in a particular subgroup of schizophrenic patients abnormalities of particular cytokines, substances with a pivotal role in immunity. They suggest that an autoimmune process is going on in these patients. The fact that, in this case as well, the observation did not hold for all schizophrenia patients is significant. In Chapter 6.2 we argued that "schizophrenia" is an invalid concept. Heterogeneity of recognised psychiatric disorders is a paramount factor that slows down progress in research on mental illness. Heterogeneity is also important in major depression. Rothermundt *et al.* (2001) observed changes in cytokines in major depression, but the changes were not the same in melancholic and non-melancholic patients. For bipolar disorder (manic depressive illness), preliminary findings also implicate cytokine abnormalities (Su *et al.,* 2002), and Kokai *et al.* (2002) suggest that such abnormalities characterise mental illnesses in general. However, observed immune responses are not the same in different mental illnesses. For example, Rief *et al.* (2001) observed differences between depression and somatisation syndrome. Several authors found changes not only in chemically mediated immunity, but also in cell-mediated immunity; recent studies suggest that cells of the immune system play a role in the pathogenesis of major psychiatric disorders (Muller *et al.*, 2000, and Nikkila *et al.*, 2001: schizophrenia; Schwarz and Chiang *et al.*, 2001: serious disorders in general; Frank *et al.*, 2002: depression).

Researchers attending the expert meeting on psychoimmunology, Innsbruck, 2000 (contributions published in Sperner-Unterweger *et al.*, 2001) confirmed the essentials of all these findings. Their contributions also show that the study of the immune system in mental illnesses is difficult. The heterogeneity of categories such as "major depression" and "schizophrenia" does not allow of easy generalisations. Furthermore, psychotropic drugs such as antidepressants and antipsychotics influence the immune system. Thus, it is difficult to distinguish between drug artefacts and symptoms of illness. The influence of stress on the immune system should also be taken into account. For example, hospitalisation may be stressful and alter immune function, so that impaired immunity need not always be a sign of mental illness *per se*. These intricacies notwithstanding, the available data converge overall to confirm the assumption that immunity plays a role in mental illness.

The findings concerning immunity add to indirect evidence indicating that omega-3 PUFAs are important in mental illness. The evidence is rich and varied. There is no denying that we have here a plausible integrative theory in the making.

10.5. The Issue of Causal Significance

We imagine that some representatives of mainstream psychiatry would respond in the following way to our line of reasoning about omega-3 fatty acids. Many causal factors play a role in the aetiology of mental illnesses. Some causes are more significant than other causes, and we have to identify the most significant ones. Processes in the brain should have primary significance, since they are intimately associated with mental phenomena and behaviours. These processes are ultimately regulated by genetic factors, the most fundamental causes. Environmental factors do play a role, but these factors are modifiers, not primary causes of mental illnesses. If omega-3 PUFAs affect the illnesses, then they belong to the category of modifiers; they cannot be root causes.

We have two responses, one about the organisation of current biomedical science, the other concerning the notion of causal significance. The existing organisation of biomedicine around genetics and molecular biology is one-sided. The idea that genetic factors have a primary role in the genesis of organismic features, whereas the environment is a source of secondary, modifying influences, is odd in the extreme. Factors in the two categories play equally important roles. We would turn the argument about genetics on its head. As omega-3 deficiencies are common and appear to cause psychiatric disorders, we may as well argue that the illnesses ensue from an environmental root cause, inadequate food, and that genetic modifiers may alter the expression of the illnesses.

Considering causal significance, we grant that many factors involving the brain (and many other somatic factors) have potential causal roles in mental illnesses. But ecological factors, psychological factors, and social factors also play causal roles. The comparative significance of particular factors will be different in different cases. If you get into a severe depression after the loss of your job, the factor of job loss is causally more significant than changes in your neurotransmitters, which no doubt will ensue. And the best treatment, if feasible, would be securing a new job rather than pills that dull your sense of job loss.

The study of aetiology in psychiatry may also get on the wrong track if the search is overmuch for causes that are special to *mental* illness. Comorbidity of psychiatric disorders with all sorts of somatic diseases is common. Horrobin (2001) suggests that this points at shared mechanisms. He argues that an impaired fatty acid metabolism caused by enzyme abnormalities plays a significant role both in mental and in somatic pathology. Thus, omega-3 PUFAs represent a promising treatment option in psychiatry (Horrobin, 2002). But Horrobin (2001) does not allot a major aetiological role to dietary deficiencies of omega-3 PUFAs. In view of the overall evidence concerning dietary omega-3 deficiencies (see Chapter 7, sections 3 and 4) we conjecture, contrary to Horrobin's view, that dietary deficiencies are indeed important in mental illness.

In brief, we single out omega-3 PUFAs as a factor that potentially has major causal significance in the entire domain of psychiatry, indeed medicine, for the following reasons. First, evidence in the form of data and theories indicates that deficiencies of omega-3 PUFAs in our diet are widespread. Second, the evidence shows that this is an important risk factor in many different diseases. Third, we can explain this since we know about biological functions of these PUFAs. We conjecture that few other factors have now as much causal significance in mental illnesses. But in specific cases, of course, the deficiencies may be irrelevant. It is to be hoped that our diets become more adequate, so that the deficiencies will lose their impact.

10.6. A Survey of the Evidence

As indicated in Chapter 7.3, eicosapentaenoic acid (EPA) and docosahexaenoic acid (DHA) are crucial among the omega-3 PUFAs. Shortages of these acids in our diet are pronounced. Omega-6 PUFAs are also important, but shortages of these acids are not as much in evidence. Moreover, the *relative* quantities of omega-3 *versus* omega-6 are important. We are getting too much of omega-6 PUFAs compared to omega-3 PUFAs (see, however, Horrobin, 2000, and Horrobin *et al.*, 2002, who disagree with this).

Quantitative relationships between omega-3 PUFAs and antioxidants also affect our health. Omega-3 PUFAs in large quantities impair our health, but this effect is counterbalanced by antioxidants. Antioxidants are a group of chemicals that counteract negative effects of free radicals, highly reactive substances liberated in our body in particular biochemical pathways.

Mahadik *et al.* (2001) and Yao *et al.* (2001) have proposed that schizophrenia is a free radical disease, in which cell membranes are damaged by an excess of these substances. They suggest that this calls for treatments with antioxidants and particular PUFAs. This is an example of yet another possible cause for schizophrenia (see comments on biological psychiatry in Section 3). But in this case the connection with diet is made so as to establish a more plausible overall picture. Conceivably, the excess of free radicals observed in schizophrenia patients may be a secondary result of inadequate diets, but medication could also have this effect. Khan *et al.* (2002) and Arvindakshan *et al.* (2003) managed to separate out confounding effects of medication. They confirmed the abnormalities of free radicals and PUFAs in schizophrenia. A comparison of drug-naive patients, patients on antipsychotics, and controls, showed that the abnormalities are not a medication artefact.

The complexity of our biochemistry precludes the feasibility of a single PUFA treatment scheme for psychiatric disorders. It warns us against rash interpretations of research on the treatments. Here is an example. Horrobin *et al.* (2002) found that EPA has beneficial effects in schizophrenia. Remarkably, a low dose of 2 g/day worked better than a higher dose of 4 g/day. The low dose was associated with higher quantities of arachidonic acid (AA), a physiologically important omega-6 PUFA in cell membranes. This finding contradicts the common assumption that omega-3 PUFAs have positive effects by enhancing AA depletion of cell membranes. Such contradictory findings are by now a familiar thing: Processes in our bodies depend on many contextual factors. Thus, we must take care to avoid sweeping claims. The results of Horrobin *et al.* also show that negative findings in experimental PUFA treatments need not imply that the treatments are no good. The dose may have been wrong, and the proper dose may depend on contextual factors. Such intricacies notwithstanding, the evidence accumulated until now does indicate that omega-3 PUFAs are a promising treatment option in psychiatry. We review hereafter a representative sample of evidence in brief.

Treatment effects have been investigated in various types of study. In the first place, we have RCTs (see comments at the end of Section 1). Most RCTs concerning serious illness have been done with patients on medication, so that PUFAs in combination with medication were compared with medication alone, the medication being regarded as a placebo. These studies mostly yielded positive results, but exceptions exist. At the other end of the spectrum of possible set-ups we have single case studies, some of which have been done with patients not receiving drugs. Common opinion has it that such studies have little evidential force. As we will argue later, we do not agree. We consider RCTs first.

Mellor *et al.* (1995) did a study with patients suffering from schizophrenia who were being treated with antipsychotics. They noticed that symptoms of the patients improved if they were treated with fish oil, which is rich in omega-3 PUFAs, in addition to the antipsychotics. The so-called positive symptoms (symptoms such as hallucinations) ameliorated and side effects (tardive dyskinesia: involuntary movements due to prolonged treatment with antipsychotics) improved. The chances are that the positive symptoms are in part an artefact caused by medication rather then a symptom of a disorder. If so, then the fish oil was redressing an inadequate treatment that was being continued. For details, see Healy (2002), reviewed in Chapter 6.3. The investigators also studied the fatty acid composition of membranes of red blood cells from the patients. Fish oil caused an increase of omega-3 acids and a decrease of omega-6 acids in the membranes. This explains the benefits of fish oil: It appears to remedy membrane insufficiencies caused by inadequate diets.

The beneficial effects of EPA added to medication in schizophrenia were confirmed in other studies (Laugharne *et al.*, 1996; Peet *et al.*, 1996; Assies *et al.*, 2001; Emsley *et al.*, 2002). A meta-analysis of four studies from the Cochrane Library (Joy *et al.*, 2001) provides additional confirmatory evidence. According to the analysis, preliminary data look promising for fish oil. EPA appears to have a moderately positive effect in schizophrenia and it may well be an acceptable intervention. A study on major depression resulted in similar findings (Edwards *et al.*, 1998). In this study as well, patients were treated with fish oil added to a common medication regime of antidepressives.

The studies indicate that a shortage of omega-3 PUFAs in cell membranes contributes to mental deterioration both in schizophrenia and in major depression. The shortage may well be due to inadequate diets (but Horrobin, 2001, in a study of depression, suggests that an enzyme deficiency may be a more significant cause, with diet as a modifying factor). Patients suffering from schizophrenia or from depression appear to respond well to omega-3 PUFAs, but the results obtained do not constitute a coherent picture. For example, since the fatty acids ameliorate depression, a natural assumption would be that they should likewise ameliorate negative symptoms rather than positive symptoms in schizophrenia. Negative symptoms such as flattened affect, unlike positive symptoms such as hallucinations, resemble depression. However, Mellor and colleagues obtained the opposite result. We conjecture that medication artefacts explain the discrepancies (see again Healy, 2002).

Some details of a study by Peet and Horrobin (2002) on the effects of an EPA-derivative in schizophrenia are remarkable. These investigators studied patients who were given different antipsychotics, alone or in combination with the EPA-derivative. EPA had positive effects if added to some antipsychotics (compared to antipsychotics alone as the placebo), but with other antipsychotics no effects were found. Thus, it should not surprise us that other authors did not observe effects of EPA added to drugs (for example Fenton *et al.*, 2001). It is difficult to interpret this kind of discrepancy. The antipsychotics influence membranes. Should their effects be regarded as positive? We would not accept that as a generally valid claim (see Chapter 4). Perhaps they wreak havoc with membranes or other structures, perhaps EPA can counterbalance this unless drug effects are beyond repair. As it is difficult to check such things through experiments that combine EPA with drugs, we hope that treatments with EPA alone will be effectuated soon. The study by Peet *et al.* (2001) indicates that the study of such treatments is a rational option. They observed positive effects of EPA added to antipsychotic medication. In one of their trials, patients were given a choice either to continue with the antipsychotic or to leave it out. Remarkably, he effects of EPA were more positive in the latter situation. Horrobin (2002) regards lipids such as EPA as a promising new treatment option that is effective in depression and schizophrenia. He states that we badly need new treatments, as the efficacy of psychotropic drugs has not improved since they were introduced over forty years ago.

Most investigations done with fatty acids but without medication are single case studies. We regard them as singularly impressive. In Chapter 3.5 we have already analysed one of them. We argued there that the evidential force of such studies can be impressive. The usual verdict that they compare poorly with RCTs does not take into account that theories may also be a source of evidence. Several theories support the assumption that omega-3 PUFAs are beneficial (see Chapter 7, Sections 3 and 4). Furthermore, patients in single case studies have improved on a PUFA treatment where other treatments failed. The results of two single case studies described hereafter are particularly convincing as the treatment effects observed were spectacular.

Puri *et al.* (2001) describe the case of a patient who had been severely depressed for seven years, with suicidal tendencies. Conventional antidepressants had not resulted in recovery. A treatment with ethyl-EPA added to conventional medication resulted in a spectacular improvement of the symptoms, accompanied by a changed fatty acid metabolism and structural changes in the brain recorded by scans.

Su *et al.* (2001) report a case of omega-3 PUFAs having spectacular effects in the absence of conventional medication. A 30-year-old married woman with chronic schizophrenia experienced an episode of acute exacerbation of psychotic symptoms during pregnancy. As conventional medication could harm the unborn child, the woman was treated with omega-3 PUFAs only. This resulted in a dramatic improvement in all her symptoms. A significant increase of omega-3 PUFAs in the membranes of her red blood cells indicated that the fatty acids did affect cell membranes in accordance with what we know about the mechanisms of fatty acid biochemistry.

It would be foolish to deny that these single case studies represent strong evidence.

10.7. Fatty Acids, Science, and Culture

The omega-3 story presented in this chapter is more than a mere search of optimal treatments for patients with a psychiatric disorder. It implies that we have to restructure psychiatry, medicine, science, indeed our entire culture. We are serious, knowing full well that this is a strong claim.

To start with, we have some additional comments on PUFAs and psychiatric disorders. The crucial role of omega-3 PUFAs in the disorders may well extend to the entire life history of patients, including the part before birth. Much research indicates that prenatal exposures play a role in the development of schizophrenia later in life. Reviews in the book edited by Susser *et al.* (1999), for example, show that prenatal viral infections and prenatal malnutrition are risk factors for schizophrenia (for references and data concerning prenatal infections and immunity, see also Schwarz and Chiang *et al.*, 2001; Schwarz and Muller *et al.*, 2001; for viral infections as a possible cause of schizophrenia and other mental illnesses, see also Pearce, 2003).

The role of omega-3 PUFAs should lead to a new understanding of prenatal exposures. As the brain needs particular omega-3 PUFAs in large quantities, it is particularly sensitive to omega-3 deficiencies while it grows and develops, before and after birth. As for prenatal malnutrition, omega-3 deficiencies deserve special attention, since they impair the immune system and thereby increase the risk of infection.

Surprisingly, the reviews in the book by Susser *et al.* do not even mention omega-3 PUFAs. The reason cannot be that the relevant information was unavailable when the book was written. Much of it had been available for decades. The explanation is presumably that we are dealing with literatures which are substantively connected but bibliographically unconnected (see Chapter 5.1). Our suggestions concerning links between prenatal exposures and omega-3 PUFAs are indeed the main subject in a review by Clandinin and Jumpsen (1997). On the basis of a large literature, these authors argue that omega-6 and omega-3 PUFAs are requisite for brain development as they arc structural components of developing membranes. The omega-6 / omega-3 ratio in our diet influences the immune system during development. It is critical that the developing foetus obtain the correct types and amounts of fatty acids to ensure complete and proper development of the brain. An inadequate fatty acid composition of the mother's diet, or the diet of the child after birth, may lead to all sorts of diseases later in life.

These insights, if combined with materials from previous chapters, result in the following picture. Numerous people in Western countries suffer from omega-3 deficiencies over prolonged periods. This contributes to a high prevalence of chronic somatic disorders and psychiatric disorders (see Chapters 7 and 8). Since many professionals do not know about the deficiencies, patients suffering from the disorders often do not receive optimal treatments. Instead, they get drugs promoted by the pharmaceutical industry, dangerous drugs without efficacy in many cases (see Chapters 4.3, 6.3 and 8, and references in these chapters). Inappropriate drugs may indeed invite the use of additional drugs aiming to redress side effects. As we argued in Chapter 8, for example, non-steroid anti-inflammatory drugs (NSAIDs, in many cases best replaced by fish oil) often cause gastrointestinal disorders subsequently treated with antibiotics and / or antacids, which invite other side effects. NSAIDs may also cause psychiatric disorders and so enhance the use of psychotropic drugs. The prevalence of this side effect has in all probability been underestimated (Defromont *et al.*, 1999).

The drug-industry connection has even led to erroneous classifications of mental illnesses (Chapter 6.3; see also Healy, 2002), which may bias research so as to perpetuate the existing situation. Bias is also fostered by the current methodology for testing medical treatments (RCTs, Evidence-Based Medicine). This methodology is adequate only if it is supplemented with independent evidence in the form of well-confirmed theories (Chapters 3 and 7) and qualitative approaches (Chapter 9).

The mess we are in is caused to a large extent not only by the pharmaceutical industry, but also by agribusiness, food production methods, and food processing methods (Chapter 7). For an appropriate health care to materialise, we would have to change many social and economic structures of our culture.

To what extent do all these things belong in the province of psychiatry? Psychiatrists should know about omega-3 deficiencies, of course. They should also be acquainted with sources that unveil links between industries and biomedical research that lead to bias. They should know about developmental neurobiology as this discipline helps us understand effects of prenatal exposures. They should know about fatty acid biochemistry in relation to agriculture and animal husbandry. And so forth. In brief, they should be acquainted with a huge store of knowledge which nobody can oversee. That is an unreasonable demand.

As professionals in other disciplines are often in the same situation, we have to conclude that the organisation of science, pure and applied, has to change in fundamental ways. Case studies in several chapters (for example Chapter 2, 3 and 5) indicate what changes are necessary. We have to shift the balance from specialist toward more generalist approaches. Some case studies in Chapter 3 showed that, if we disregard factors such as poverty and structural violence in epidemiological studies, we get models that are false *from a biomedical point of view*. By implication, the maintenance of scientific quality requires that boundaries between disciplines have to dissolve. That is possible only by generalist work. The omega-3 story is an additional example calling for drastic changes in our culture.

Meanwhile, researchers and practitioners in psychiatry have to go on with their work, with limitations and restrictions that are not of their own making. We hope that our survey helps alter the nature of some limitations and restrictions by a shift from some drug therapies toward diet therapies.

10.8. Conclusions

1. Recent large increases in the prevalence of mental illnesses indicate that human suffering is being medicalised into illness. The medicalisation is caused to a large extent by the pharmaceutical industry, which profits by overmedication with psychotropic drugs.

2. Biological causes of mental illnesses in the form of brain abnormalities are often inferred from drug effects. That is a fallacy. This attribution of the illnesses to biological causes hampers the discovery of other causes.

3. Shortages of omega-3 polyunsaturated fatty acids (PUFAs) in our food appear to contribute to psychiatric disorders. Much indirect and some direct evidence suggests that treatments with PUFAs can be beneficial even in severe disorders such as schizophrenia. In most studies to date, the omega-3 PUFAs have been combined with psychotropic drugs. It is to be hoped that the study of treatments with PUFAs alone will get a higher priority, since the use of psychotropic drugs is often problematic.

4. The significance of omega-3 PUFAs may help us explain

many features of psychiatric disorders. They are implicated, for example, in prenatal exposures as a risk factor in schizophrenia.

5. The role of the immune system in mental illnesses is undervalued. Impaired immunity in these disorders may ensue from deficiencies in omega-3 PUFAs, and treatment with these PUFAs could often be a better option than drug treatment.

6. To come to grips with mental illnesses, psychiatry has to reckon with a great variety of cultural factors.

Chapter 11

Conventional Medicine and CAM

11.1. Introduction

Disciplines are dissolving at an ever-increasing pace. In the past we had biology and psychology, for example, with vague but recognisable boundaries. By now they have spawned offspring such as psychophysiology, psychoneuroimmunology, and many more. Similar spawnings are to be seen everywhere in science. Boundaries between offspring, if visible at all, are in a process of perpetual flux. Disciplines with clear boundaries virtually do not exist any more.

It is not to be denied that groups exist of persons who may describe themselves, for example, as psychophysiologists, and that journals often have names such as psychophysiology in their titles. But this does not mean that words such as "psychophysiology" denote entities in the real world. If such entities existed, we should be able to classify them into clear-cut individual disciplines. That is obviously impossible.

Problems with the recognition of disciplines are like problems with the recognition of diseases. It is true that some of the diseases recognised by medicine do exist in the sense that we can reliably and validly attribute them to patients by particular signs and symptoms (see Chapter 2). But other "diseases," for example schizophrenia as defined by the DSM, do not exist in this sense (see Chapter 6.2). The recognition of diseases is arbitrary in many cases. Widespread comorbidity, the phenomenon of patients suffering from combinations of diseases, indicates that nature does not contain a store of diseases as neat and orderly packages.

As arbitrariness goes into disease classifications, so does it infect classifications of disciplines dealing with disease. Consider the case of migraine (see Chapter 5). "Migraine" as a disease label represents a heterogeneous collection of diseases, each characterised by signs and symptoms with much variability among patients. What discipline could cover migraine in a faithful way? The short answer is that no such discipline exists. To understand biological aspects of migraine, we have to draw on neurology, endocrinology, anatomy, biochemistry, and so forth.

For a comprehensive understanding, we should add to this elements from psychology and the humanities.

To what extent do all these disciplines represent reality? Considering migraine, we can at most say that each of them covers some features of some patients in some situations. To come to grips with migraine, we have to integrate elements from different "disciplines," but variability among patients precludes that any integrative view should be generally valid.

This state of affairs invites the metaphor of an ideal science that functions as a supermarket. Science contains knowledge products in miscellaneous assortments. If we wish to develop it further, or apply it to some theoretical or practical problem, we may happen to come across an assortment that suits our current purposes. Thus, in some situations a ready-made assortment of knowledge from some "discipline" may help us understand a particular disease, or find a treatment for a patient. In other situations, no ready-made assortment of knowledge products may be helpful, so that we have to compose an assortment of our own from a variety of sources.

The ongoing dissolution of boundaries between disciplines could help us approach health and disease with an open-minded, generalist attitude. However, in the present cultural climate such an attitude is more easily preached than practiced, for several reasons. First, knowledge or what passes as knowledge, is generated in medicine in quantities so large that nobody can oversee even what is happening in their own specialties (see Chapter 5.1). Second, power and money are concentrated in organisations and industries with vested interests that increasingly determine the course and the content of medical research and medical treatments. Third, privileged areas of research generate one-sided approaches of health and disease. Many case studies in the foregoing chapters indicate, for example, that the emphasis in medical science is overmuch on a restrictive sort of biology.

In some areas of medicine and psychiatry, this situation has caused a decline in quality (see Chapters 4, 6, 8 and 10). That is one reason why old distinctions of conventional *versus* complementary and alternative medicine (CAM) are no longer valid. A common conception has been that conventional medicine is the most adequate source of theoretical and practical knowledge, as it draws on evidence obtained by reliable, objective methods and theories of science, whereas the methods and theories of CAM are below standard (see for example the volume edited by Sampson and Vaughn, 2000). Of course, representatives of CAM do not share this view. They argue that many CAM therapies have evidential force (for a survey, see Pelletier, 2000). But their standards of forcc are way beyond Evidence-Based Medicine. Middle-of-the road approaches envisaging bridges between conventional medicine and CAM are also being followed, but they are less common (Vincent and Furnham, 1997; Muskin, 2000). Furthermore, there are those who do not see a well-defined classification of medicine as the general public is making such a classification impossible (for all sorts of variations on this theme, see O'Connor, 1995; Gordon *et al.*, 1998; Kelner *et al.*, 2000).

We reject the dichotomy of conventional medicine and CAM. In Section 2, we reconsider limitations of conventional medicine, with implications for boundaries of medicine as a whole, and boundaries between conventional medicine and CAM. In Section 3, this is made more concrete by comments on some varieties of CAM.

11.2. Boundaries of Medicine

Disciplines are dissolving. Our metaphor of science as a supermarket explains why we welcome this development. Case studies in previous chapters indicate that tendencies in medicine to stay within strict disciplinary boundaries may result in bad theory and bad practice. The dissolution of disciplinary boundaries may improve our understanding of health and disease. By boundary dissolution we do not mean that classifications of knowledge domains must be abandoned. That would invite chaos. We can fruitfully use disciplines as ever-changing knowledge stores, but we must not take them to represent separate subdivisions of reality.

Any partition of science into disciplines is necessarily associated with a division of labour. No professional can at the same time be endocrinologist, geneticist, psychologist, and so forth. So we need collaboration among representatives of specialties, in biomedical research and in health care. Profitable collaboration is feasible only if everybody is to some extent a generalist. At the very least, they should know about main trends in potentially relevant disciplines outside their own specialty. Otherwise they would not know what forms of collaboration are feasible and desirable. We gather that few would quarrel with this, as we have been stating the obvious. But opportunities for acting on the obvious are limited in medicine. Examples in previous chapters illustrate this. We briefly look at some of them again.

The influence of diet, especially omega-3 fatty acids, on health and disease, has since long been charted outside mainstream medicine (see Chapters 7, 8 and 10). Contributions from food science, evolutionary biology and anthropology convincingly show that the average diet in "civilised" countries is unnatural and that it fosters many chronic diseases. Particular omega-3 acids used as food supplements are an invaluable asset to prevent and treat these diseases. Therapies with these acids would presumably outperform many drug therapies. Yet, the medical community has mostly ignored this. Information concerning the acids deserves to be accommodated in theories and practices of many medical specialties. Alternatively, the information could be kept within food science, but then the information should in some way spread to these specialties. Neither option has been implemented to a desirable extent.

Other examples of disciplinary boundaries drawn with unfortunate effects are to be found in Chapter 3. Tuberculosis is on the increase in some developing countries and also, locally, in developed countries (Chapter 3.3). Within medicine, epidemiologists have attributed this to multiple drug resistance of bacteria and the emergence of AIDS. Social scientists have pointed to additional causes, notably lack of patient compliance with treatments and shortcomings of health care delivery. Neither the epidemiologists nor the sociologists have realised that structural violence increases the prevalence of tuberculosis. Hence, existing views of aetiology are inadequate, as a significant cause is being disregarded. Should medical theory and medical practice be concerned, then, with the political issue of structural violence? Yes, they should or, alternatively, they have to accommodate information from other disciplines dealing with violence. Structural violence is sometimes a significant aetiological factor in tuberculosis. If it is disregarded, we get a one-sided aetiological theory and a one-sided medical practice, which may cost us dearly.

A similar story is to be told about local, aetiologically significant associations of air pollution and poverty (Chapter 3.4), and additional examples of one-sidedness in medicine are to be found throughout the book.

The examples have implications for the boundaries of medicine. The biomedical model (in a narrow sense of the term) assumes that medical science—not medical practice—should stay with biological aspects of health and disease. Adherents of this model would not deny that non-biological factors affect health and disease. Thus, they have to assume that these factors must be studied by professionals from other disciplines such as psychology, sociology, economics and politics. If needs be, theories from these disciplines could be combined with biomedical theories.

This strategy easily leads to inadequate theories. The omega-3 fatty acid story is a telling example. We could restrict research about the fatty acids to investigations of diets and their physiological effects. That would amount to plain biology, a kind of biology often disregarded in medicine, for that matter. But a really satisfactory view of diet and health must also account for causes of inadequate diets. We need to know about pervasive negative effects on our health of modern food processing done for economic reasons, and equally pervasive negative effects of unnatural feed provided to our cattle for economic reasons (see Chapter 7). Leaving these things out on the ground that they are more than mere biology, strikes us as an odd way of doing medical science. We get dangerous nonsense in this way, not only in medicine but also in economy. For example, economic cost-benefit models justifying current forms of agriculture and husbandry are unsound *economically*, if costs that accrue to health care due to bad food are omitted.

The example of tuberculosis and structural violence is another case in point. The analysis in Chapter 3.3 indicates that scientists who disregard the factor of structural violence are likely to develop theories—epidemiological theories within medicine or sociological theories outside medicine—which are *false* as they overestimate the causal contributions of other factors. In this case we need to do research that accounts for the factor of violence right from the start. Now, a defender of the biomedical model may regard this research as a combination of biomedicine and political science, and call the resulting theory of tuberculosis an interdisciplinary theory. Or the entire enterprise may be called biomedicine with elements borrowed from elsewhere. It is all the same to us as long as relevant factors are in the research project. The labels are mere terminology.

Nobody would deny that medical practice should be more than applied biology. But as our examples indicate, medical science should not be restricted to biological approaches either.

11.3. Conventional Medicine, CAM, and Culture

Disciplines are entities with an elusive sort of existence. That much is clear by now. Boundaries drawn between medicine and other domains of science, indeed culture, have to depend on the context, and they are always arbitrary to some extent. We can but expect that the same situation exists in complementary and alternative medicine (CAM). Indeed, the definition of CAM has been a source of perpetual controversy and confusion. Most disputes about conventional medicine *versus* CAM presuppose that CAM is ill-defined, whereas conventional medicine is well-defined. This dividing line is misleading as conventional medicine is not well-defined either.

Once we decide that medicine confined to biological approaches will not do, we run the risk that its floodgates open onto an indefinite multitude of disciplines concerned with health and disease. We obviously cannot allow the entire multitude to pass the floodgates. How, then, are we to identify approaches that may enrich biomedicine? This question is unanswerable as it is misconceived. It has us look from disciplines to phenomena rather than the other way round. Phenomena of health and disease should be our first concern. Any selection of disciplines, or theories, or kinds of professionals, is best adapted to concrete concerns. If as a result of poor sanitation, drinking water in a city is polluted with bacteria causing an epidemic, then medical professionals in the city will have to know about it. This is not to say that they have to take responsibility for, say, the funding of better sanitation. That kind of thing is now in the domain of other professionals. Thus, divisions of labour define the boundaries of medicine in the case at hand. The divisions of labour derive from culture, not nature. They are ultimately a matter of political choice.

Back to the dichotomy of conventional medicine and CAM. Moyad (2001) presents a clear analysis of definitional problems with CAM. His concern is with medical practice; he does not consider theories and worldviews associated with CAM. We comment on two passages that represent common views in conventional medicine.

Moyad notes that CAM seems to encompass "alternative medicine" or "integrative medicine" or "unconventional medicine" or "non-traditional treatments" or even "unproven therapy."

> In reality, it [CAM] should ideally include those interventions that have been adequately tested in basic science and clinical studies. Although, if an intervention or treatment has been adequately tested, then it would theoretically not be considered "alternative." Rather ... it would be a part of the field of medicine or the field of conventional medicine. Alternative seems to imply those treatments that contain no evidence. (Moyad, 2001: 257)

Implicit in this passage is the assumption that interventions in conventional medicine "have been adequately tested in basic science and clinical studies." Many examples in our book show that this assumption is not generally valid. Moyad would presumably grant this. Hence, we take him to mean that "conventional medicine" stands here for "good conventional medicine," to be distinguished from "bad conventional medicine."

To make Moyad's distinction of conventional medicine and CAM workable, we have to know the meaning of the key terms "adequately," "tested," "basic," and "science." Moyad presents a list of CAM therapies which includes, for example, herbal medicine, folk remedies, lifestyle diet and homeopathy. He suggests that, barring some exceptions, such therapies have not yet been adequately tested with positive results. "Tested" appears to refer to methods such as clinical trials, "adequacy" obviously concerns positive outcomes of such trials. We assume that "science" is not restricted here to biology. If it were, then many "alternative" therapies, if proven effective, could not be accommodated in conventional medicine as they are associated with different areas of science. But from this interpretation, we are at a loss to understand the word "basic," which appears to point in a different direction.

We are in sympathy with Moyad's remarks, but we would like to turn the tables on conventional medicine itself. The use of standard methodologies in conventional medicine has been criticised by many researchers (see Chapters 4, 6, 8 and 9). Randomised controlled trials (RCTs) are beset with methodological pitfalls. In conventional medicine, these pitfalls are often disregarded, with the result that many RCTs violate elementary methodology. Also, many drug therapies in conventional medicine are problematic owing to roles of the pharmaceutical industry (see Chapters 6, 8 and 10).

More fundamentally yet, regarding evidence in conventional medicine that does support some therapy, we may rightly comment in many cases: It is evidence, but evidence of what? The answer that the therapy works well with a particular disease will not do. It is altogether too general. For example, RCTs as a source of evidence are performed under specific conditions, with patients that have to satisfy all sorts of criteria. So the evidence can only support the claim that the treatment works well in a restricted setting. The very rigor of tests may make them artificial in that they do not allow extrapolation to real life situations, which are complex and "messy" (see Chapters 4, 6, 8 and 9).

In brief, when we opt for a particular methodology in conventional medicine, we always pay a price for it. Rigor may for example decrease realism. Representatives of CAM would often opt for more realism and less rigor. This invites the following characterisation. Evidence in favour of conventional treatments may be strong while being somewhat out of touch with relevant domains of application. Evidence in favour of alternative treatments may be weak while being more in touch with relevant domains of application. In either case, the approach chosen may satisfy methodological criteria of science, but with different priorities. We simply cannot comply with all the criteria at the same time. Hence, the dividing line between conventional medicine and CAM cannot be a straightforward matter of evidence. Evidence is always evidence relative to criteria, and a uniform application of criteria would be undesirable, if it were possible at all.

The distinction of conventional medicine and CAM becomes even more problematic if theories and worldviews are taken into account. Research articles in conventional medicine that address the distinction, like the article by Moyad, almost always focus on treatments. The assimilation by conventional medicine of "proven" treatments from CAM by no means implies that underlying theories of CAM would be assimilated as well. If we do account for the theories, we get a distinction of the two domains of medicine that does not sit well with Moyad's view. Many CAM theories, for example those of acupuncture, cannot be accommodated by present-day conventional medicine. But it would be unwise to divorce such theories entirely from the treatments associated with them. The treatments are informed by the theories, and they are assumed to confirm them. Conceivably, treatments may be beneficial even if the theories underlying them are false. Such a situation is common, for example, with psychotherapies (see Chapter 4.4). The matter is important, because theories are a potential source of evidence (see Chapters 3.2, 4.2, 7.3 and 10.4).

It is understandable that researchers in conventional medicine do not like to bother about, for example, "subtle energies" as postulated by adherents of many schools of CAM. The notion of "subtle energy," for persons schooled in Western modes of thinking, is intolerably vague and unclear. But so are notions such as "psychogenic" (Chapter 2.3) and "placebo" (Chapter 4) in conventional medicine. The issue at stake concerns relations between the mental and the physical. Conventional medicine does not have a generally accepted theory about these relations. If it sticks with the physical in the form of biology, then it is bound to miss essential aspects of health and disease. We applaud the signs that conventional medicine and CAM may be able to realise convergences of treatments, but these would only represent one step on the way toward a more integrative medicine. As yet, some worldviews found in CAM, particularly CAM with an old non-western tradition, cannot be assimilated by conventional medicine for lack of a shared language (see for example the book on traditional Chinese medicine by Kaptchuk, 2000, who presents a detailed analysis of the problem).

While professionals on both sides pursue better theories and therapies, we should not forget about the role of laypersons. Moyad

(2001), in another telling passage, implicitly suggests that they do not have expertise which counts:

> If a treatment was found to enhance the results of conventional therapy ..., then it could probably be termed "complementary." If a treatment was found to improve the prognosis for a patient by itself, then it could probably be termed a "conventional treatment" ... . Ideally, it seems that after appropriate research has been completed, "complementary" may just encompass those therapies that patients are able to provide for themselves after instruction or encouragement from the appropriate health professional is given. (Moyad, 2001: 257)

We wonder what Moyad would think about "therapies that patients are able to provide for themselves" *without* "instruction or encouragement from the appropriate health professional." Should treatments within the grasp of laypersons be kept outside the domain of medicine?

Folk medicine has in store for us lots of valuable, simple treatments (but also a lot of rubbish) (see Chapter 3.1). If known in the population at large, it would be odd if we consulted medical professionals about the treatments. This invites a new perspective on the boundaries of medicine. To the division of labour among different professionals, which as we saw affects the boundaries of medicine, we have to add a division of labour for professionals *versus* laypersons. The existing emphasis on biology in medicine suggests that we should rework the former division of labour. The existing medicalisation of society suggests that we need to rework the latter division of labour also.

11.4. Toward a Reappraisal of CAM

The literature about CAM is large and bewildering by its heterogeneity. We consider samples from two multi-author volumes, Vickers (1998) representing views within CAM, and Fontanarosa (2000) representing studies of CAM in conventional medicine. The views expressed in these volumes are also to be found in more recent articles. As they are representative, we have not included additional references.

The Fontanarosa volume contains reprints of articles in high-ranking medical journals, most of which appeared in 1998. It was published by the American Medical Association (AMA), with a critical but positive approach. As in the previous section, we argue that the demarcation of conventional medicine in general from CAM in general does not serve us well.

The two volumes illustrate a point made in the previous section. The representatives of CAM in the Vickers volume have much to say about theories and worldviews associated with treatments, but the AMA volume is almost entirely devoted to treatments alone.

The Vickers volume is remarkable as the contributors, many of them practitioners of CAM in the United Kingdom, have set themselves to the task of self-criticism. They are aware that a critical attitude is often rare in their professions. In the words of the editor: "Turn to just any book on complementary medicine and you will usually be hard pressed to find even a single statement that criticises any theoretical or practical aspect of the therapy concerned" (Vickers, 1998, Introduction: 2). Worse, "Certain professional groups have actually enshrined their opposition to critical evaluation in codes of practice" (idem: 3). Vickers identifies several factors that contribute to this situation. The practitioners often engage in outward criticism of conventional medicine as they have to maintain a position outside of it, they often miss criticism as they work alone, they mostly rely on a tradition that venerates a founding figure, and they have to defend themselves against attacks.

Criticism from opponents of CAM has been harsh. Vickers shows that the opposition often fights CAM with unfair advocacy and politics rather than objective science. The well-known volume edited by Stalker and Glymour (1989) and publications of so-called "sceptics" illustrate this. However, the tides may be turning. Representatives of conventional medicine are aware that CAM has by now a huge share in the health market, and also that some CAM therapies might become a valuable addition to conventional therapies. But they will insist that CAM should be subjected to critical tests, preferably RCTs.

Kaptchuk and Eisenberg (1998), in the Vickers volume, analyse the history of alternative dietary lifestyles. They show that dietary reform movements are typically led by lay people who claim to be able to understand nutritional science. Until recently, the biomedical literature has branded the movements as "fads" or "cults" or "quackery," with the implication that they are transitory phenomena, but this overlooks their having been a persistent and enduring part of the health care scene for almost 200 years. The movements come in many kinds, but they share three core beliefs: nature as a guideline, vegetarianism, and the conviction that dietary reform is essential in the rehabilitation and regeneration of society. This variety of CAM obviously has significant moral and ethical overtones. Kaptchuk and Eisenberg note that conventional and alternative views of nutrition have lately come closer to each other, but differences remain as dietary reform movements continue to carry overtones of a moral crusade.

For an assessment of research on diet, nutrition, lifestyle, and herbal therapies, we turn to the AMA volume. Goodwin and Tangum (2000) have an interesting contribution about micronutrient supplements. They observe that the medical community has long opposed, and often still opposes, the idea that deficiencies of micronutrients may be an important cause of ill-health.

> Negative attitudes about micronutrients did not evolve recently; they have deep roots. The resistance of the medical community to the concept that scurvy, beri-beri, and rickets were caused by vitamin deficiencies has been well documented. ... But the pathologists who dominated academic medicine in the late 19th and the early 20th centuries lacked the vocabulary to integrate the public health observations of vitamin deficiency into a pathophysiology dominated by the germ theory. (Goodwin and Tangum, 2000: 219)

A telling example mentioned by the authors is the thesis of the Nobel laureate Pauling that micronutrients such as vitamin C in levels above minimum requirements are beneficial (see Chapter 7.2). This is now a respectable hypothesis—not a well-confirmed one—but 20 years ago is was regarded as quackery. They end the article with a lesson from history:

> Ideally, issues such as the theory underlying the treatment or the guild to which the proponents of the treatment belong should be irrelevant to the fundamental questions of efficacy, toxicity, and cost. The history of the response of academic medicine to micronutrient supplementation suggests that we have not attained that ideal. (Goodwin and Tangum, 2000: 220)

Health food movements may obstinately oppose diets that do not fit with the strong moral convictions they have. Conventional medicine does not exercise this kind of opposition, not in the same degree at any rate. But opposition without a valid scientific justification exists here as well. Human beings often cling to cherished ideas, and scientists are no exception.

The AMA volume has 23 contributions on herbal therapies.

Together they show that promising therapies exist alongside therapies which are presumably worthless. As with conventional drug therapies, side effects, even dangerous ones, may occur, and interactions between conventional drugs and herbs may also cause problems. Numerous patients use herbs, and many thousands of preparations exist. Yet, we have no adequate regulation for their use, and scientific evidence of their efficacy is limited as the pharmaceutical industry has no incentive to investigate herbs for lack of patentability.

All in all, a critical assessment of the entire therapeutic landscape is practically impossible. But we can aim to investigate particular preparations deemed potentially significant in view of frequent usage, or provisional folk evidence, or information about pharmacologically active components. Herbs are in principle a rich source of new medications. They always have been in conventional medicine. Thus, no reason exists to relegate them to a separate domain called CAM.

The problem that we are unable to gather all the information needed to asses existing treatments is even worse than the example of herbal therapies already indicates. With herbs, we have the problem that the available information is a tiny fragment of what we need to know. At least as severe is the problem that information which *is* available often cannot be managed by us if it reaches us at all (see especially Chapter 5).

Considering diet and food supplements, one of us (WJS) illustrates the information problem with some autobiographical comments on omega-3 fatty acids as available in fish oil. Evidence from many sources presented in Chapters 7, 8 and 10 demonstrates that deficiencies in these acids are common, that they contribute to diseases and disorders in "civilised" countries, and that fish oil often helps remedy deficiencies in a preventive or even curative fashion, more so than drug therapies in many cases. Millions of people could benefit from this. But the medical community is slow to recognise this, and the existing balance of power does not favour the replacement of drug therapies by diet therapies, if appropriate (cf. roles of the pharmaceutical industries and governmental agencies, reviewed in Chapters 8 and 10).

During the last decade, I (WJS) have been in touch with many persons in The Netherlands about this problem. Here is what I found out. In athletics, amateurs and professionals have known about fish oil for a long time, their diet being an important factor affecting performances. Druggists I met also knew about it. Some of them were able to inform me about fatty acid biochemistry in relation to health. I have also put the matter before a number of biologists. With them I often got the response that they were sceptical, as they had never come across the subject in standard texts of biochemistry or physiology. Some of them commented that the matter belongs to medical research, which is to be distrusted anyway as medicine is not science. Responses from officials advising the government were remarkable. One of them did not wish to air public comments on policies concerning drug therapies *versus* diet therapies for fear of getting out of work. The other official was to advise the government about the therapies. He indicated that existing shortcomings of policies could not be mentioned in an official advice for political reasons. Instead, the emphasis should be on the prevention of future shortcomings. Teachers at one of the best colleges of alternative medicine we have, most of them practitioners also, knew all about the omega-3 fatty acids. But unless diet was their specialty, they did not have them as a formal item in their treatment repertories or their teaching, since they regarded the matter as so elementary that everybody should know about it. Lastly, I have been in touch with several physicians and psychiatrists about the drugs *versus* diets problem. Until recently, I was told by persons in this category that what I was telling them could not be true. If it were, then they should have heard about it. But during the last year some of them reported that the fish oil story is catching the attention of the medical community. Several psychiatrists indicated that the omega-3 story has been in recent conferences, and that they take it seriously. I was also told that omega-3 treatments of psychiatric patients have to be done in combination with drug treatments, as the pharmaceutical industry is funding the research. Some psychiatrists also commented that general practitioners prescribe psychotropic drugs (where fish oil might be more effective) in large quantities, against the consensus in psychiatry that this practice is irresponsible. One psychiatrist told me that his profession had years ago given up militating against this situation, since previous actions had been fruitless. These autobiographical notes are not hard evidence, but they suffice to indicate that we have to improve on existing flows of information.

The two volumes we are considering do not contain information about fish oil. We continue our survey with interesting pointers from a sample of articles about two areas of CAM, traditional Chinese medicine (TCM) comprising herbal therapies and acupuncture, and homeopathy.

Birch (1998) presents in the Vickers volume an impressive overview of acupuncture traditions. He demonstrates that schools of acupuncture have existed for 2,000 years, that an impressive variety of schools has developed in different social and political climates, and that many of those writing about acupuncture do not know about the existing diversity.

Despite the ready availability of evidence of

> diversity in acupuncture, most commentators make more limited descriptions which they then use as if they applied to the whole field. (Birch, 1998: 50)
>
> Investigators thus run the risk of investigating things that may be inaccurate, and, in particular, that cannot be generalised. Examples can be found in the clinical trial literature, where inadequate knowledge of the practice of acupuncture has fostered assumptions about what constitutes an adequate treatment, and thus what should be an appropriate control treatment ... . Faulty assumptions ... usually lead to very poorly conceived notions of what should constitute a 'sham,' 'placebo' or 'control' needle treatment. (Birch, 1998: 56)

During the last decade, many RCTs have been done to assess the efficacy of acupuncture, with mixed results. Birch's comments indicate that the real work has yet to be undertaken.

The inadequacies of research seen by Birch are aggravated by limitations shared by all RCTs (see Chapters 4, 6, 8 and 9). Particularly relevant is a point which we have been making throughout the book: The very rigor of RCTs entails a restricted validity of outcomes, as they apply only to the conditions prevailing during the trials. We therefore need precise descriptions of settings in which particular variants of acupuncture are being tested, and RCTs should not be our sole source of evidence. For example, single case studies can be an important source of evidence if their outcomes get support from other sources (cf. studies of schizophrenia described in Chapters 3.2 and 10).

From the AMA volume, which has several articles about acupuncture, we take an interesting single case study. Nasir (2000: 495-496) describes the case of an acupuncture consultation sought by an internal medicine service for a 25-year-old woman who had been re-admitted only hours after having been discharged from a 4-day hospitalisation for treatment of severe migraine. Several medications had been tried, all without relief. The woman had been suffering from migraine for many years, and she had been treated in several clinics without much change in the headache frequency or severity. She was sceptical about acupuncture, but consented to be treated. The headache resolved within one hour of treatment, and she slept soundly through the night, with only a mild return of the headache the next morning. A second treatment resolved the headache, and she remained free of symptoms afterwards while being treated as an outpatient.

At the very least, this study invites more research on acupuncture. The evidence that acupuncture worked in this case is not absolutely compelling; no evidence ever is. But it is not to be dismissed lightly for being anecdotal. In principle, the outcome may be explained without the assumption that the acupuncture treatment worked. But the fact that other treatments had not worked adds credence to this assumption. It deserves to be counted as part of the evidence. We need many more accurate, detailed case studies like this one. They could result in a kind of cumulative evidence that is now rare, since large-scale studies with conceptually homogenised patient populations have become the measure of research on treatments in conventional medicine.

Alongside acupuncture, herbal therapies have always been a stock in trade of TCM. The Vickers volume has no contribution on herbal TCM. Koo and Arain (2000), in their contribution to the AMA volume, review many studies of this treatment mode. Although most studies had not been well designed, the evidence as a whole suggests that promising herbal treatments exist in TCM. But it is difficult to test the treatments, as TCM practitioners often prescribe mixtures of many herbs, so that effects cannot be attributed to particular components. Furthermore, the composition of herb mixtures may show much variation, and dangerous side effects have been noted.

The most convincing study is by Bensoussan *et al.* (2000) in the same volume. They conducted a double-blind RCT of herbal therapy applied to irritable bowel syndrome (IBS), noting that, to their knowledge, theirs was the first clinical trial fully adhering to TCM. They studied two treatments, a standard TCM treatment for all patients in one group, and an individualised treatment in which the herbs administered were chosen to fit characteristics of individual patients, in another group. Outcomes in both groups compared favourably with outcomes in the placebo group, with few side effects.

This case study is encouraging as 10 to 20 per cent of the population in the United States and Australia suffer from IBS (for references, see Bensoussan *et al.*, 2000). We have a caveat, though. The authors call IBS a functional disorder (for comments on this notion, see Chapter 2.4). They apparently assume that the causes of the disorder are unknown, and they state that no available treatment has been reliably effective; the patients use a variety of approaches for symptom management, including drugs, dietary modifications and counselling. This description is a telling example of *MSA* (missing stuffs and arrows; see Chapter 1) as it omits vital information. One of us (WJS) has done a study of the disorder which uncovered information that is missing here. It was published in Van der Steen and Thung (1988: 48-50). We briefly summarise the essentials.

Halfway through the 1980s, I (WJS) knew a patient suffering from IBS. She was a very stable personality. Yet, specialists in internal medicine all came with the advice: Go see a psychiatrist. Many patients at the time were being treated in this way as IBS was indeed regarded as a "functional" disorder. However, I discovered that research in the United Kingdom had since long shown that IBS may be caused by multiple food allergy with impaired immunity. Volumes with all the details had already been published in the United Kingdom. Moreover, a Swiss double-blind study had shown that the drug sodium-cromoglycate may effect a cure. This drug was then used to treat asthma. (An immunologist recently told me that it is now regarded as a treatment of choice for multiple food allergy.) I informed the general practitioner treating the patient about the literature I had uncovered, and he was flabbergasted. Nobody had ever told him about it. I got the same response with several learned specialists of internal medicine.

At the time, other therapies were also known to be effective, most notably elimination diets. But these therapies were then prescribed only by doctors who had also specialised in "alternative" medicine. The elimination diet strategy was tried out by the patient, and she got well in a short time.

We conjecture that other types of diet therapy may also work well with IBS, as dietary deficiencies are implicated in many chronic disorders. Omega-3 fatty acid deficiencies are common (see Chapter 7), and they affect the immune system—which is impaired in IBS. Therefore, we would like to see research on the effects of fish oil on IBS. The efficacy of the TCM treatment may also involve the immune system; this is another point to be investigated. Anyhow, to arrive at the best treatment of IBS, we first of all need to have all available information at our disposal, from "conventional medicine" and from "CAM." The example of IBS confirms that existing flows of information are inadequate.

Homeopathy is the last variety of CAM considered here. The basic theory of homeopathy was developed by Hahnemann in the late 18th century. He formulated its central principle, *similia similibus curentur*, or like cures like. The idea of the central principle is that a substance which produces particular symptoms in a healthy human being, can cure the same symptoms in a sick human being. Substances are tested by a procedure called proving, in which symptoms in healthy volunteers are observed and recorded. Homeopathic drugs are mostly used in high dilutions prepared by a process called potentisation. High potencies may not even contain a trace of the active substance. Its activity is assumed to carry over to the solvent. This has been a cause for much ridicule among opponents of homeopathy. However, recent research suggests that preparations might work even at high dilutions. (See, however, Merrell and Shalts, 2002, whose list of methodological shortcomings in ongoing research looks devastating. We would comment that the shortcomings are common also in conventional medicine.) Some homeopaths avoid high potencies. The work of Mössinger (1984) in Germany is an example. He argues that potentisation does not make sense, while aiming to integrate conventional medicine and homeopathy. Unfortunately, as far as we know, his view has failed to get a foothold in the Anglo-Saxon world.

Much literature suggests that homeopathy has a coherent tradition with a single theory, and one cumulative store of prescriptions based on provings. The actual situation is not at all like that. Swayne (1998), in an overview in the Vickers volume, demonstrates that homeopathy is commonly misrepresented. He shows that it is characterised by much diversity of theories, philosophies underlying the theories, prescribing strategies, actual prescriptions, doses and potencies, and *materia medica* and repertories (which contain information about medications related to symptoms). Yet, if attitudes of patients are a measure of success, homeopathy does very well.

> The evidence in every country where homeopathy is practised is that patients feel better for it however we do it. This is the worrying thing. This is the ultimate ground of scepticism. If people get better whatever we do, does it actually matter what we do? It is commonly said in conventional medicine that a multiplicity of treatments for any one condition is a measure of how little benefit any of them provide. In homeopathy, whose patients often choose it because of the limitations of conventional treatments—and claim benefit from it, the problem is slightly different. If all of them work, do any of them really work? (Swayne, 1998: 70-71)

Worse is to come. In the same volume, Fisher (1998) analyses the evidence on which homeopathy is based. According to its own criteria, much of it is inadequate. Provings are often flawed. Moreover, one of the most important sources, Kent's repertory, is problematic since "we have no idea who observed which symptoms to be cured in which disease under what circumstances. This information appears to have been lost, if, indeed, it was ever recorded" (Fisher, 1998: 80). In practice, homeopaths seldom follow the precepts they are supposed to work with. They use new, formal methods of matching medications with symptoms, and often rely on experience and information exchange with colleagues. All in all, it is hard for us to assess existing evidence.

The AMA volume contains several articles about homeopathy. One of them (Weiser *et al.*, 2000) is a promising study of vertigo. The authors used a homeopathic preparation which had been successful on previous occasions, and compared it with a conventional medication, betahistidine, in a double-blind RCT. The outcomes demonstrated that the two treatments are therapeutically equivalent. We do hope that this kind of work will become more common. Also, we would like to see more scrutiny on the side of conventional medicine of single case studies in homeopathy. As indicated in our comments on acupuncture, such studies may be a valuable supplement of RCTs with their inherent limitations.

Considering possible merits and demerits of CAM, we would not pass a general judgment. Valuable CAM treatments appear to exist alongside treatments that had better be rejected. This is also true of conventional medicine. As we have indicated throughout this chapter, we would like to witness the dissolution of boundaries between conventional medicine and CAM. Good medicine exists alongside bad medicine, in conventional medicine and in CAM. The challenge for the future is for us to find as many locations as we can where gems of good theorising and good practice may lie in wait for us.

11.5. Conclusions

1. The classification of scientific knowledge into disciplines is arbitrary to a large extent. Likewise, conventional medicine and complementary and alternative medicine (CAM) are ill-defined entities, neither of which covers all significant aspects of health and disease. It may be wise to stop aiming at any fixed demarcation of conventional medicine and CAM.

2. The organisation of knowledge is best adapted to concrete undertakings. If our concern is with deficiencies of omega-3 polyunsaturated fatty acids (PUFAs) in our diet, we need to know about fatty acid biochemistry, food processing and cattle feed, for example. This information, however heterogeneous, yields a coherent perspective on relations between diet and health. To come to grips with relations between structural violence and tuberculosis, or relations between air pollution, poverty and disease, we need different combinations of elements from science and culture at large.

3. Concrete undertakings in medicine call for a generalist attitude

and common sense. Biology would not suffice as a scientific foundation for medicine.

4. A generalist attitude is also necessary for spotting lacunae in research, and distortions of existing approaches, in conventional medicine and in CAM. An analysis of particular approaches in CAM, for example acupuncture and homeopathy, reveals much variability among schools which is often disregarded by commentators and analysts.

5 CAM therapies are being tested in conventional medicine, in some cases with positive results. But theories of CAM are seldom considered in conventional medicine. It is to be hoped that bridges between conventional medicine and CAM are going to extend from therapies to theories and worldviews.

Chapter 12

Medicine and Religion

12.1. Introduction

When you enjoy eating an apple pie, physical processes in your brain and elsewhere in your body are associated with the emotion of enjoyment. Without the eating and the pie, the processes would not be there, or they would be different. Knowing that it is an apple pie you are eating is likewise associated with brain processes in some way. Scientists would not be capable to identify the processes down to details that match your emotions and cognitions. But they would be confident on good grounds that the processes must exist, and they may even manage to describe them in general if not detailed ways.

Few persons would deny that such associations between mental processes and physical processes exist. Yet, the nature of the associations is an enigma as the mental and the physical appear to represent utterly different domains of reality. Over centuries, science and philosophy have had in stock a variety of incompatible theories about the enigma. Ever since the philosopher Descartes (1596-1650) put forward his dualistic mind-body theory, the nature of "the mind" and "consciousness" in relation to the body has remained a vexing problem (see for example the accessible survey by Bechtel, 1988, the critical analysis of theories by Seager, 1999, and the anthology edited by Block *et al.*, 1997).

The view of Descartes has been branded as unintelligible, since it postulates a "ghost in the machine" without a clue of how ghosts and machines could interact. Thus, few researchers nowadays defend dualism in the spirit of Descartes. But modern variants of his views do exist (see for example Nelkin, 1996). Different views come in many varieties. Some researchers defend the unvarnished view that mental phenomena are in fact no more than the behaviour of nerve cell assemblies and their associated molecules (Crick, 1994). Others regard this kind of identification as simplistic because the "reduction" of the mental to the physical should be more intricate (Kim, 1998), or because we have to accommodate the environment in theories relating the mental to the physical (Clark, 1997). Some theorists assume that networks of "dumb" nerve cells are able to generate complex processes experienced by us as mental (Bechtel and Abrahamsen, 1991). Next, we have numerous theories that relate particular mental phenomena to processes in the nervous system without much "deep" philosophy, in the so-called cognitive neurosciences (see the multi-author enterprise edited by Gazzaniga, 2000). All these trends are dismissed by philosophers who take an analysis of ordinary language as their point of departure (McClintock, 1995). Philosophers in the ordinary language tradition attribute the problem of the ghost in the machine to a kind of linguistic confusion.

Over and above controversies about all these theories, we are saddled with disputes about the very feasibility of adequate theories. Some defend the view that such theories are impossible, because we cannot understand consciousness owing to limitations of our cognitive capabilities. Others regard the problem of consciousness as almost solved (see the articles edited by Shear, 1997, which represent opposing views). Anyhow, attempts to reach consensus about particular fundamental theories of the mental and the physical have been a dismal failure, and the signs are that the failure is going to stay with us for a long time.

Considering everyday problems of health and disease, we regard all the abstract philosophical literature as singularly unhelpful. Indeed, in view of the chronic nature of the disputes, we conjecture that the entire undertaking is on the wrong track. Therefore, we would not plead for any general theory of the mental and the physical. In biomedical research and in medical practice, we often manage to deal with relations between the mental and the physical without bothering overmuch about general philosophy. The example of the apple pie indicates that we do not need a sophisticated mind-body theory to find out about concrete interactions between, say, emotions and hormones.

In previous chapters, we did steer away from general mind-body philosophy without getting into trouble. However, the subject of the present chapter, medicine and religion, calls for a more overt philosophical stance. We approach the subject by mundane, open-minded analyses of texts and cases that do touch on philosophy, but we keep avoiding abstract philosophy.

Would it be possible for biomedical science to justify religious worldviews? In Section 2, we contrast two opposing views of the issue while developing a pragmatic approach of our own. In Section 3, we approach the more specific theme of near-death experiences (NDEs) in the same spirit.

12.2. Opposing Views

Processes in brains are nowadays studied with techniques called neuro-imaging or brain imaging. The techniques involve sophisticated machines that make images of the processes visible in a literal sense (see Uttal, 2001, for details and critical comments). The machines could be used to generate images of processes taking place in your brain while you are eating an apple pie. In a way, the *brain* images would represent what is in your *mind* as you deal with the pie. No consensus exists about the nature of the representation. Indeed, the very notions of "representation" and "mind" are metaphors for things that defy full understanding.

Metaphorically, your dealings with the pie are in your mind, and the images of the brain processes confirm that what is happening in your mind is also represented in your brain. Now, it would be odd to assume that the pie exists *only* in your mind and in your brain. The pie experienced by you exists also as a thing before you on the table, as long as you have not eaten it, that is.

People may also experience things that exist without being as concrete as the pie in the example, or experience things that do not exist at all. For ease of exposition, we refer to the two (admittedly heterogeneous) categories of experiences as *perceivings* and *imaginings*, respectively. We also use the italicised words *perceive* and *imagine* in line with this.

Throughout the ages, many persons, great mystics in particular, have reported that they have experienced God. The expression "experiencing God" is to be taken here as a metaphor used in keeping with other metaphors such as "being united with the cosmos." The experiences belong to the realm of religion or, more broadly, spirituality, which lies nowadays beyond the domain of mainstream science with its materialistic flavour (for diverse views in the philosophy of religion concerning the implications of the experiences, see for example Forman, 1990; Evans, 1993; Guthrie, 1993; Carmody and Carmody, 1996; Gellman, 2001). Many scientists confronted with such reports, would regard the experiences as *imaginings* rather than *perceivings*, or they would merely hold that science has to treat them as *imaginings*, or they would simply regard this as a matter beyond science.

The passage quoted hereafter is from a book by two scientists (and a journalist participating in the writing) who during many years have investigated experiences of "God" ("mystical," "transcendental," experiences) by recordings with neuro-imaging techniques of brain activity in persons who are meditating (Newberg *et al.*, 1991).

> ... our experiment with Tibetan meditators and Franciscan nuns showed that the events they considered

> spiritual were, in fact, associated with observable neurological activity. In a reductionist sense, this could support the argument that religious experience is only imagined neurologically, that God is physically "all in your mind." But a full understanding of the way in which the brain and mind assemble and experience reality suggests a very different view.
>
> Imagine, for instance, that you are the subject of a brain imaging study. As part of this study, you have been asked to eat a generous slice of homemade apple pie. As you enjoy the pie, the brain scans capture images of the neurological activity in the various processing areas of the brain where input from your senses is being turned into the specific neural perceptions that add up to the experience of eating the pie: olfactory areas register the delightful aroma of apples and cinnamon [and so forth]. The ... brain scan would show all this activity in the same way that it revealed the brain activity of the Buddhists and the nuns, as blotches of bright colour on the scanner's computer screen. In a literal sense, the experience of eating the pie is all in your mind, but that doesn't mean the pie is not real, or that it is not delicious. (Newberg *et al.*, 1991: 36-37)

Newberg *et al.* had demonstrated by extensive research that in mystical states of consciousness, a particular area of the brain is activated. This should not come as a surprise. No doubt, we are capable to influence our physiology by altering states of consciousness, as in meditation. Correlations between religious experiences and physical phenomena should indeed exist as *all* mental processes have to be accompanied by physical processes in some way.

The point of interest is how we interpret the correlations. Do reports from meditators and mystics about their religious experiences merely convey what they *imagine*, and that they are deluded if they maintain to have *perceived* realities beyond ordinary awareness? The argument in the passage quoted indicates that the data from neuro-imaging are compatible with the existence of religious *perceivings* in addition to mere *imaginings*. It does not constitute evidence in favour of *perceivings*.

Newberg *et al.* (1991: 107-113) develop by additional arguments a religious worldview with Buddhist affinities. They criticise the view that mystic experiences are on par with derangements as seen in mental illnesses. According to them, the experiences of mystics are utterly different for example from those of psychotics. This seems to be a valid point, but we must exercise some caution. Oliver Sacks has interesting cautionary comments on the visions of the famous mystic Hildegard von Bingen (12th century), which are special as she described them in great detail and even left pictures (see Chapter 5.9). According to Sacks, the visions strikingly resemble particular auras experienced by some migraine patients, which could (not necessarily should) be interpreted as *imaginings*. Many other authors have also suggested that parallels exist between religious experiences and brain-based abnormal experiences in mental illnesses (for example Saver and Rabin, 1997). Persinger (1987) has shown that religious experiences during epilepsy seizures resemble similar experiences induced by the stimulation of a brain area (the temporal lobe) that plays a role in the seizures. The philosopher Churchland (2002: 381-389) comments that this kind of evidence counts against religious worldviews, although it is not compelling. This kind of evidence is important. But attempts to explain all religious experiences as mental aberrations ensuing from pathology would strain credulity.

In the last chapter of their book, Newberg *et al.* develop a comprehensive worldview that postulates an Absolute Unitary Being as an ultimate reality, more real than the material world and our subjective awareness of self. Their arguments are logically akin to the reasoning in the passage quoted, which does not have much evidential force. But the authors do not pretend to have proved anything. They only aim to argue that "the existence of an absolute is at least as rationally possible as is the existence of a purely material world" (idem: 155). That looks like a reasonable, open-minded stance.

An intriguing article by Chibmall *et al.* (2001) provides a nice contrast with the view just discussed. These authors do not aim to reach the realm of the religious by way of science. On the contrary, even though they are positive about science while also representing three different religions (Catholicism, Judaism and Protestantism), they regard attempts to forge substantive connections between science and religion as misguided.

The subject of their article is effects of distant intercessory prayer on disease. They originally intended to study the subject through experiments of their own. But upon extensive reflection they came to the conclusion that the undertaking would not make sense, for methodological reasons and also for theological reasons. The authors criticise existing literature on the subject, which in their view is methodologically flawed. We omit an analysis of the flaws, some of which could be remedied. More important is the thesis of the authors that methodologically sound studies are theoretically impossible.

Their main focus is on prayer involving God. They hold that God cannot be a subject of research as God is per definition beyond the realm of science. That may be so in the context of the religions they represent. In the context of Buddhism, we would have a different situation (see the foregoing discussion of the book by Newberg *et al.*).

In passing, the authors declare that their arguments would apply to research on distant healing in general. Thus, what they have to say also concerns a variety of alternative medicine that need not involve prayer in a narrow sense.

The most important point in the article concerns the validity of concepts. We quote some passages illustrating the point.

> But what are the critical dimensions of the construct *prayer*? Prayer, by definition, is "an address or petition to God or a god in word or thought." But what else matters?
>
> The list we generated [in thinking about an experiment to be undertaken] began as follows: Is the amount of prayer important? Is the type of prayer important? The form? The duration? [And so forth.] (Chibmall *et al.*, 2001: 2529)

It is obviously impossible to explicate the notion of prayer in such a way that studies on effects of prayer could comply with canons for, say, randomised controlled trials (RCTs) designed to test medical treatments.

> The very concept of prayer exists only in the context of human intercourse with the transcendent, not in nature. (...)
>
> Consider an analogy. A clinical trial is planned to study the effect of antibiotic agents on a new strain of respiratory bacteria. The investigators go to great lengths to ensure random assignment, placebo control, and double-blinding (as did our distant intercessory prayer researchers). But this is not all they go to great lengths to ensure. They control the type of antibiotic, the dose of the antibiotic [and numerous other things]. Why? Because all these factors are critical to the construct validity [construct = theoretical concept] of the cause; that is, they are part of the definition of "antibiotic." [We cannot interpret results unless we care

> for such details.] No model guides our understanding of intercessory prayer as a treatment in the way we know that drug pharmacokinetics, type, dose, schedule, interactions, and treatment length are critical to an antibiotic as a treatment. In fact, we believe no scientific model can guide it. (Chibmall *et al.*, 2001: 2530)

The authors subsequently argue that prayer cannot be accommodated in theories that presuppose mechanistic causality, and that we cannot test hypotheses concerning prayer as we cannot derive test implications from them. We are capable of finding effects in studies of prayer. But, the authors argue, such effects are meaningless because it is impossible to get them into a methodologically sound theory of natural science. In brief, they are arguing against the view that *supernatural* entities or forces can be accommodated in natural science.

Religion may influence health and disease, and this influence can be studied, for example, with methods of epidemiology. The authors readily grant this (for additional information and references, see for example Lewis, 2001, who shows that the issue is complex as effects of religion may be positive in some respects, and negative in other respects; according to several recent studies, the evidence in favour of any effects is weak; see for example Sloan *et al.,* 1999; Sloan *et al.*, 2000; Mueller *et al.*, 2001; Sloan and Bagiella, 2002). The authors also grant that medical practice has to take note of religion: Religious dimensions of suffering are deserving of consideration in humane interactions between doctors and patients. But theories of medicine and religion have to stay apart: "We do not need science to validate our spiritual beliefs, as we would never use faith to validate our scientific data" (idem: 2535).

The main point made by Chibmall *et al.* concerns the validity of concepts. We agree with them that concepts which have become entrenched in science should be valid in that they must have a foothold in the real world known to us. That is why we had better dispense with the concept of schizophrenia, for example. It does not even remotely have such a foothold (see Chapter 6.2). We also agree with the authors that the concept of prayer, if linked with the "supernatural" right from the start, has no such foothold either, albeit for different reasons. But we can choose to bracket connotations concerning the supernatural, and investigate "natural" aspects of distant healing (broadly defined, possibly including religious aspects in some sense of the term). As a matter of fact, distant healing is investigated in this way. Evidence suggests that it may well be effective, but as yet it is inconclusive (for a review, see Ebneter *et al.*, 2001). Studies of intercessory prayer in particular also suggest that healing at a distance is possible, but in this case as well, the evidence is not very strong (Koenig, 2001; Pearsall, 2001).

We do not accept the antibiotics analogy of the authors for two reasons. First, the test of antibiotics concerns a highly specific example of medical treatments. Research concerning other treatments need not call for detailed specifications of experimental conditions as the authors list. Furthermore, the authors are mistaken in regarding such conditions as part of the *definition* of the antibiotic; the mistake, which is known as operationism, has been exposed as such more than half a century ago in the philosophy of science (for comments and examples, see Van der Steen, 1993a: 22-23).

Second, the authors argue that a concept, to be valid, has to be accommodated in an established model or theory of natural science. The antibiotics example satisfies this requirement, whereas distant healing in general and intercessory prayer in particular fail on this count. However, the case of distant healing concerns phenomena which are *new* in the context of conventional medicine. How could they ever get a foothold there, if they should concur with established models or theories right from the start? If that were a reasonable methodological requirement, we would never be able to achieve scientific progress.

The autobiographical example from one of us (WJS) that follows illustrates the rationale of our objections. I (WJS) once woke up with a severe backache. A friend of mine knew about it, and I knew about activities of hers that may be regarded as distant healing. After I had been working for hours in a library, about five miles from the place where my friend resided, I had an odd, unfamiliar experience. It felt like a snap in my back. Concurrently, the backache disappeared instantaneously. Being a methodologist, I noted the time to the minute, and I searched for a hypothesis that could explain the phenomenon. This is what I came up with: My friend was doing distant healing in focusing on my back with an attitude of love. When I met my friend later on, I asked if she had focussed on my aching back. She answered in the affirmative. I asked if she had noted the time. She had. The time noted by her appeared to correspond with the time noted by myself, to the minute. Many more examples like this one are known to me.

The example concerns anecdotal evidence. That is a weak point. The hypothesis contains vague elements. That is also a weak point. However, from the hypothesis I had inferred a precise prediction of the time at which my friend had focussed on my back. The prediction was verified. That is a strong point. At the very least, we have here a phenomenon that calls for further investigation. If similar cases would be confirmed, the phenomenon, however defined, deserves to get a place in science, even though existing theories of *conventional* science cannot explain it.

Should we assume that future developments of science will have to accommodate such phenomena by new theories, say, of physics? We have no idea. The assumption is anyhow vague as we do not know what the new physics required for this should look like. For myself (WJS), the example involves a "force of love" associated with a "religious" attitude.

Enough of this. We do not wish to write about personal "religious" convictions. Our example shows that some aspects of phenomena such as distant healing can be approached with sound methods of empirical science. If the phenomena happen to have religious aspects in some sense of the term, we may aim at a view that combines "scientific" aspects and "religious" aspects. Or we may find that such a combination would not serve any purposes we have. Unimportant in either case would be the precise meanings of "science" and "religion" as general categories. Such overarching categories do not have visible boundaries in reality.

12.3. Life and Death

> *As she left the tunnel, familiar footholds in reality dissolved into experiences unlike anything known to her. The tunnel had been familiar as it was entirely dark. Like everybody else, she knew about the varieties of darkness, real in a forest at night, metaphorical in depressed moods induced by vagaries of life. Entirely unfamiliar was the bright, white light beyond the tunnel in which she now bathed. A voice with resonance of love then came with a clear message. "Go back to your unfinished business with cherished ones on earth. Not yet are you allowed to be with those who passed the threshold known to you as death." Longing she felt at seeing far away the shapes of relatives and friends who had died before her own time. The vision faded. Sucked she was, back into her bruised body. Then she remembered. The accident, the emergency room, doctors operating on her, seeing it all as if she floated somewhere near the ceiling, hearing a nurse say that she was a goner. And then the tunnel, the light, the voice, the dead alive and well. A goner she was not. Back to the grind mills of the earth. Much later would she come to feel that aversions to life's darker vagaries*

> *had lost their hold on her, as traces of the light stayed with her like memories of the future.*

A nice fairy-tale, that is how some would characterise this story. We have composed it as a common denominator of some tales of persons who came near death. What they experienced goes nowadays by the name of near-death experiences, NDEs for short. Experiences of being elsewhere, outside the body, are known as out-of-the-body experiences, OBEs for short. In previous publications (Van der Steen and Thung, 1988; Van der Steen, 2000c) one of us has briefly commented on these phenomena. The analysis in the present section is more detailed, and more up to date. We begin with a brief summary from the section about NDEs in Van der Steen (2000c).

NDEs and OBEs associated with them are a subject of intensive research characterised by deep controversy. Some researchers consider NDEs as a foretaste of afterlife, others regard them as hallucinations induced by brain impairment. The latter view is defended with vigour, for example, by Blackmore (1993). She argues that the tunnel vision is caused by lack of oxygen and excess carbon dioxide in particular areas of the brain. According to her, neurological processes in the brain subserving perception, explain features such as the tunnel and the white light experienced by persons having an NDE. Feelings of happiness and well-being attending NDEs cannot be explained in this way. But we can accommodate them as well under the explanatory umbrella of biology: They may be caused by the release of particular substances, endorphins, in the brain.

On the basis of such analyses, Blackmore rejects religious interpretations. Logically, her explanations are compatible with religious interpretations. But, Blackmore argues, they do weaken religious claims. She grants that paranormal phenomena in NDEs, if confirmed, would weaken her own view. But she did not uncover any convincing account of such phenomena. Some reports suggest that subjects provided accurate observations of events that took place while they were apparently unconscious. Blackmore assumes that such observations are residual perceptions under apparent unconsciousness.

Blackmore also presents an integrative scientific theory that in our view weakens her case. From cognitive science she borrows the theory of mental models. During NDEs, she argues, our normal models of self and world break down so that we lose contact with reality. The same happens, for example, during meditation, when we lose the sense of self.

> So my proposal is quite simple: that the system

> [that I am] takes the most stable of its models and attributes to it the status of "real." Our "reality" at any time is the brain's collection of stable mental models built largely out of sensory input and integrated to form a model of self in the world. It is, if you like, a "me-now model." It describes me and my place in an apparently real world.
>
> And is there a real world out there? Well, if we adopt this view we can never know. We assume there is in the way we talk about brains and what they do. But it is only an assumption—a useful working model. (Blackmore, 1993: 161)

Blackmore argues that normal, stable mental models ensue from adequate sensory information. Failing this information, as in NDEs, the models break down, so that information from stored experience gets the opportunity to induce hallucinations and illusions.

This line of thinking appears to be self-defeating. On the one hand, Blackmore endorses neurobiological explanations that treat our experience of self as an illusion. The self is merely a mental model that dissolves in experiences such as NDEs. On the other hand, Blackmore's view has to entail that the deliveries of neurobiology are also mental models that may represent illusions.

Here is an alternative analysis that turns the tables on Blackmore's view. Under particular conditions, as in meditation, our mental models dissolve so that we are capable to recognise the illusions of science for what they are. NDEs represent rare phenomena which unveil realities that are unavailable in normal awareness, because mental models, for example those delivered by neuroscience, obscure these realities from our perceptions.

Many of those who, unlike Blackmore, believe that religious experience tells us something deep about reality, would agree with her that the world of appearances is an illusion. But contrary to Blackmore they would hold that mystical experiences rather than materialistic science unveil reality beyond appearance. Blackmore flatly denies the existence of such a reality. But her line of reasoning awkwardly implies that the denial ultimately draws on illusions. The summary from Van der Steen (2000c) ends here.

We appear to have reached a stalemate. *Imaginings* or *perceivings?* That is the question (see the previous section). Meanwhile, we have to consider that this dichotomy may in a way be misleading. What kind of entity should it be who *imagines* or *perceives* phenomena beyond realities created by conventional science? Under meditation, during NDEs, and in states described by mystics, the ordinary sense of self and personhood lose meaning as boundaries between the individual and the world dissolve. Ordinary language and the language of science cannot adequately express what is happening then.

The stalemate is to be found in many other writings dealing with NDEs. An entire issue of the *Journal of near-death studies* (Vol. 16, number 1, 1997) is devoted to it. Jansen (1997), in the opening target article, defends the view that brain biochemistry may suffice to explain NDEs. He argues that ketamine, a psychoactive substance, induces experiences resembling NDEs. This substance acts on the neurotransmitter glutamate by blocking a receptor for it, the N-methyl-D-aspartate receptor (NDMA receptor for short).

Six critical comments follow the article by Jansen. We quote some representative passages from the target article and from one of the other articles, by Fenwick (1997), with a running commentary.

> There is overwhelming evidence from thousands of studies relating brain events to alterations in mental state that "mind" results from neuronal activity. The dramatic effects on the mind of adding hallucinogenic drugs to the brain, and the religious experiences that sometimes result, provide further evidence for this ... .Within the scientific paradigm, it is not possible [to assume that the spirit leaves the body, leaving a brain with its sensory functions intact]. (Jansen, 1997: 6)

Comment. "Within the scientific paradigm," indeed. But the paradigm is the very issue at stake.

> Attempts to explain the NDEs as hallucinations are sometimes rejected by spiritualists because many persons insist upon the reality of their experiences ... . However, 30 percent of normal subjects given ketamine were certain that they had not been dreaming or hallucinating, but that the events had really happened ... . (Jansen, 1997: 10)

Comment. Perhaps the events did happen. According to the scientific paradigm endorsed by Jansen they are out of bounds but, to repeat, the paradigm is the very issue at stake.

> Any physician dealing with head injury, epilepsy, or altered cerebral physiology knows that as cerebral function becomes compromised it becomes disorganized. Even in such simple circumstances as ordinary fainting, recovery from the faint is recovery from a confusional process. Acute cerebral catastrophes result in confusion and not clarity. This important fact is overlooked by those attributing simple chemical explanations to the NDE. Although ketamine may produce experiences that are similar to the NDE, and Jansen has argued cogently that it does, he does not explain how these same experiences can arise in a dysfunctional brain. His argument is that when brain processes have been so disorganized that there is loss of consciousness, consciousness can then be resynthesized in its clarity by a brain mechanism such as flooding the brain with NMDA inhibition. Surely the very fact that consciousness has been lost would argue that cortical activity is insufficient to sustain high quality and clear consciousness as would be required for an NDE (Fenwick, 1997: 45-46).

Comment. Fenwick rightly notes that the evidence with which Jansen defends his worldview is weak. He points to the feasibility of a very different worldview:

> Turning now to the nature of mind, Jansen quoted the standard identity theory, which states that brain processes are entirely responsible for, and identical with, subjective experience. In other words, he presented the standard scientific view ... . However, one of the interesting and exciting points about the NDE is that it suggests that our view of mind may be too limited. It raises the possibility that mind may be *nonlocal*. Nonlocal means that although brain processes within the skull are involved in the structuring of mind, the effects of mind may extend beyond the brain. (Fenwick, 1997: 49) [Next, Fenwick cites sources from parapsychology and NDE literature providing anecdotal evidence of genuine OBEs.]

Comment. This is a superficial summary of views found in New Age literature that uses quantum mechanics to support spirituality—an odd combination of bedfellows. The argument derails here. The expression "nonlocal" is at odds with "extend beyond," which presupposes location. We again come here across the problem that some phenomena can hardly be formulated in the language of current science. Fenwick apparently holds this view as well, as the end of his article indicates:

> One is left only with the subjective accounts. Science, by definition, cannot explain subjective experience, so it can neither refute nor confirm the possibility that these subjective accounts do indeed suggest that some form of personal experience may continue during the unconsciousness of brain catastrophe or even after brain death. (Fenwick, 1997: 52)

This is a fallacy with the following structure: "*A* has the subjective experience that *B* occurs; we cannot explain the phenomenon of subjectivity; therefore: we cannot check whether *A* has the subjective experience that *B* occurs." It is indeed true that we have no easy means to check all the things reported about NDEs. But some things can be checked. Patients who experienced an OBE during surgery may report not only about the tunnel and all that, but also about the surgery itself, or about a traffic jam on the road alongside the hospital. A test which confirms that such things occur would support the hypothesis that "some form of personal experience may continue during the unconsciousness of brain catastrophe or even after brain death." The test would also lend some support to the more outlandish aspects of NDEs, albeit in remote, indirect ways. But this kind of support is normal and acceptable even in sophisticated science. Straightforward, direct links between evidence and fundamental theories are rare if they exist at all.

The opposing views we described illustrate the persistence of the stalemate that characterises much NDE research. To overcome the stalemate, we need a broader perspective on the phenomena and the data before embarking on theorising. The most comprehensive surveys known to us are to be found in the books by Kellehear (1996) and Fox (2003). Here are some items from Kellehear's book, which covers extensive areas of science and culture.

- Non-Western NDEs are very different from Western NDEs. Many researchers disregard significant information about non-

Western NDEs that does not fit with their theoretical predilections.

- Many features of NDEs are also present in situations of danger but good health and normal conscious awareness. So linking them with impending clinical death is misleading.

- One-sided reports of researchers foster popular conceptions of NDEs as providing glimpses of a world beyond this one, or an afterlife.

- The forms taken by NDEs and similar experiences are influenced by cultural factors and by the social experiences of the person.

- Generalising descriptions of NDEs that refer to tunnels and suchlike, often derive from interviews, or correspondence, with leading questions inviting the use of particular words, for example "tunnel." If persons who had the experiences tell about them without being pushed to use prefabricated language, we get stories with an extensive variability. The variability is suppressed in all current theories.

- The materials used by some leading researchers are biased as they are used used in selective ways.

- The assumption that those who approach the issue from within "modern" science, for example neuroscience, are operating in an objective, value-neutral mode, is demonstrably false. Their articles are full of rhetorical devices, dogmas and insinuations. If you develop an eye for this, the matter becomes shockingly obvious.

The last point is particularly important, because it is easily overlooked in science (see also Zingrone, 2002, who made the same point in her presidential address for the Parapsychological Association).

The bias found in "modern" science with its emphasis on neurobiology, and bias in NDE reports reinforce each other. Fox (2003), in an extensive analysis of case studies, confirms Kellehear's view that generalising descriptions of NDEs are not to be trusted. He also shows that neurobiological explanations, for example the explanations offered by Blackmore and Jansen, miss the mark as they misrepresent the phenomena to be explained. NDEs do share some features, experiences of darkness and light for example, but features explained by the neuroscientists do not in fact characterise most NDEs. The explanations have many additional shortcomings. Thus, they do not in any way accommodate the narrative features of NDE reports.

Fox also criticises religious "explanations" that use reports of OBEs to posit the existence of a soul that can leave the body. The evidence that persons having an OBE did reliably perceive events elsewhere is weak. We describe hereafter the most striking case study known to us, by Sabom (1998), reviewed and put in context by Greyson (2000: 339-340). We have not been able to check up on details of the case; Fox does not mention it. If it is methodologically impeccable, then it has far-reaching implications.

A woman had to undergo a dangerous type of brain surgery that necessitated the temporary interruption of physiological processes without which we cannot normally survive. This can be done at body temperatures way below the normal range. A considerable risk to do this was taken in the case of the woman, as the alternative of doing nothing was even more risky. Being in this situation during some 45 minutes, the woman was dead, as it were. Her brain was devoid of electrical activity (formally: brain death), since blood had been completely drained from it. Also, she had a prolonged cardiac arrest during this period and had to be shocked to restore blood circulation in the rest of the body.

Afterwards, the woman reported to have been out of her body, observing from above the entire procedure, the persons involved and their activities, and much more, in great detail. The details of her report showed a perfect fit with the situation actually existing while her brain could not have functioned in any way recognised by medical science.

However we may choose to explain this phenomenon, it would stick out like a sore thumb if put into the shopping basket of materialistic prophets of neuroscience. When forced to make the choice, we would prefer souls to thumbs.

12.4. Conclusions

1. Mystical experiences have correlates in the brain. The correlation implies nothing about the veridicality of the experiences. Some do claim that they may reveal deep truths about God or the cosmos. This claim is way beyond the evidence. Others reject the very possibility that research could provide information about religious truths, or *vice versa.* Their view is overly pessimistic. In between these extremes, we should be

able to do research that may redraw existing boundaries between science and religion.

2. Near-death experiences (NDEs) have particular significance in the study of religion related to medicine. Incompatible extreme views exist in research about NDEs. Some regard NDEs as a window on afterlife. Others explain them as products of brain malfunctioning. The evidence produced by adherents of either view has visible shortcomings. Further research about NDEs may well force us to revise fundamental assumptions of biomedicine and science in general.

Afterthoughts

In closing, we feel like revisiting the woman facing an icy river. We slightly change the story as told in Chapter 9.2:

> Imagine a woman standing by an icy mountain river, intending to cross to the other side. A team of four risk assessors stands behind her, reviewing her situation. *They know about a bridge upstream, but they decide to ignore it. Their assignment is to assess situations in a limited area where they happen to meet the woman, and the bridge is outside this area. Here is what they say to the woman.*
>
> The toxicologist says that she ought to wade across the river because it is not toxic, only cold. The cardiologist says she ought to wade across the river because she looks to be young and not already chilled. Her risks of cardiac arrest, therefore, are low. The hydrologist says she ought to wade across the river because he has seen other rivers like this and estimates that this one is not more than 4 feet deep and probably has no whirlpools at this location. Finally, the EPA policy specialist says that the woman ought to wade across the river because, compared to global warming, ozone depletion, and loss of species diversity, the risks of her crossing are trivial.
>
> The woman refuses to wade across. "Why?" the risk assessors ask. They show her their calculations, condescendingly explaining to her that her risk of dying while wading across the river is one in 40 million.
>
> Still, the woman refuses to wade across. "Why?" the risk assessors ask again, frustrated by this woman who *refuses to act on their advice*.
>
> The woman points upstream and says "Because there is a bridge." (O'Brien, 2000: 3; italicised passages ours).

The original passage from O'Brien's book (2000) was a starter to reveal that prevailing Evidence-Based Medicine is incomplete. Evidence-Based Medicine is a powerful tool for answering questions about health and disease. It is not a tool for finding the right questions. We have shown that the questions asked are often wrong. Medicine is not to be blamed for this in all cases. True, it often failed to ask the right questions about subjects in its domain, in the case of diet for example. But other unasked questions are outside its domain as usually defined, questions about the impact of poverty and political abuse on health and disease for example. We have to redraw the boundaries of medicine to get such questions on the agenda.

The modified passage from O'Brien concerns a more serious matter. However odd and outrageous, it becomes realistic if we draw an analogy with Evidence-Based Medicine adapted to agendas of persons and organisations with vested interests in the health market. Known truths about medical treatments are often withheld from us, and false claims about medical treatments are not as rare as they should be.

The situations we described are a cause for moral concern. Yet they are seldom seen on the agendas of ethicists in general and medical ethicists in particular. We have refrained from allotting an explicit role to ethics in our book, but our moral stance should by now be obvious. We can but hope that purified roles of medical knowledge are going to materialise through a democracy that generates a new morality.

References

Abraham, J. (1995), *Science, politics and the pharmaceutical industry: controversy and bias in drug regulation.* London: UCL Press.

Abraham, J. (2002), 'The pharmaceutical industry as a political player', *Lancet*, 360: 1498-1502.

Abraham, J., D. Bardelay, C. Kopp, J.D. Kleinke and E. Bennion (2002), 'Education and debate: Making regulation responsive to commercial interests: streamlining drug industry watchdogs', *British medical journal*, 325: 1164-1169.

Addae-Kyereme, J., S.L. Croft, H. Kendrick and C.W. Wright (2001), 'Antiplasmodial activities of some Ghanaian plants traditionally used for fever/malaria treatment and of some alkaloids isolated from Pleiocarpa mutica; in vivo antimalarial activity of pleiocarpine', *Journal of ethnopharmacology*, 76: 99-103.

Albert, C.M., H. Campos, M.J. Stampfer, P.M. Ridker, J.E. Manson, W.C. Willett and J. Ma (2002), 'Blood levels of long-chain n-3 fatty acids and the risk of sudden death', *New England journal of medicine*, 346: 1113-1118.

Albino, A.P., G. Juan, F. Traganos, L. Reinhart, J. Connolly, D.P. Rose and Z. Darzynkiewicz (2000), 'Cell cycle arrest and apoptosis of melanoma cells by docosahexaenoic acid: association with decreased pRb phosphorylation', *Cancer research*, 60: 4139-4145.

Alcaraz, A., and J. Kelly (2002), 'Treatment of an infected venous leg ulcer with honey dressings', *British journal of nursing*, 11: 859-866.

Alexander, J.W. (1998), 'Immunonutrition: the role of omega-3 fatty acids', *Nutrition*, 14: 627-633.

Allen, C., M. Bekoff and G. Lauder (eds.) (1998), *Nature's purposes: analyses of function and design in biology.* Cambridge, Massachusetts:

MIT Press.

Almallah, Y.Z., S.W. Ewen, A. El-Tahir, N.A. Mowat, P.W. Brunt, T.S. Sinclair, S.D. Heys and O. Eremin (2000), 'Distal proctocolitis and n-3 polyunsaturated fatty acids (n-3 PUFAs): the mucosal effect in situ', *Journal of clinical immunology*, 20: 68-76.

Appenzeller, O. (1991), 'Pathogenesis of migraine', *Medical clinics of North America*, 75: 763-789.

Ariza-Ariza, R., M. Mestanza-Peralta and M.H. Cardiel (1998), 'Omega-3 fatty acids in rheumatoid arthritis: an overview', *Seminars in arthritis and rheumatism*, 27: 366-370.

Arvindakshan, M., S. Sitasawad, V. Debsikdar, M. Ghate, D. Evans, D.F. Horrobin, C. Bennett, P.K. Ranjekar and S.P. Mahadik (2003), 'Essential polyunsaturated fatty acid and lipid peroxide levels in never-medicated and medicated schizophrenia patients', *Biological psychiatry*, 53: 56-64.

Ashford, N.A. (1999), 'A conceptual framework for the use of the Precautionary Principle in law', in: C. Raffensperger and J.A. Tickner (eds.), *Protecting public health and the environment: implementing the Precautionary Principle.* Washington, D.C.: Island Press, 198-206.

Assies, J., R. Lieverse, P. Vreken, R.J. Wanders, P.M. Dingemans and D.H. Linszen (2001), 'Significantly reduced docosahexaenoic and eicosapentaenoic acid concentrations in erythrocyte membranes from schizophrenic patients compared with a carefully matched control group', *Biological psychiatry*, 49: 510-522.

Assouad, M., S.L. Vicks, M.V. Pokroy and R.J. Willcourt (1994), 'Recurrent acute interstitial nephritis on rechallenge with omeprazole', *Lancet*, 344: 549.

Backer, M., D. Sander, M.G. Hammes, D. Funke, M. Deppe, B. Conrad and T.R. Tolle (2001), 'Altered cerebrovascular response pattern in interictal migraine during visual stimulation', *Cephalalgia*, 21: 611-616.

Ballesteros-Amozurrutia, M.A. (2000), 'Peptic ulcer and *Helicobacter pylori*. Results and consequences of its eradication' [Spanish], *Revista de gastroenterologia de Mexico*, 65, Supplement 2: S41-S49.

Bandyopadhyay, D., K. Biswas, M. Bhattacharyya, R.J. Reiter and R.K. Banerjee (2001), 'Gastric toxicity and mucosal ulceration induced by oxygen-derived reactive species: protection by melatonin', *Current molecular medicine*, 1: 501-513.

Banks, W.A., A.J. Kastin, and S.I. Rapoport (1997), 'Permeability of the blood-brain barrier to circulating free fatty acids', in: S. Yehuda and D.I. Mostofsky (eds.), *Handbook of essential fatty acid biology: biochemistry, physiology, and behavioral neurobiology.* Totowa, New Jersey: Humana Press, 3-14.

Bannwarth, B., E. Dorval, A. Caekaert and P. Barthelemy (2002), 'Influence of *Helicobacter pylori* eradication therapy on the occurrence of gastrointestinal events in patients treated with conventional nonsteroidal antiinflammatory drugs combined with omeprazole', *Journal of rheumatology*, 29: 1975-1980.

Barber, M.D. (2001), 'Cancer cachexia and its treatment with fish-oil-enriched nutritional supplementation', *Nutrition*, 17: 751-755.

Barber, M.D., K.C. Fearon, M.J. Tisdale, D.C. McMillan and J.A. Ross (2001), 'Effect of a fish oil-enriched nutritional supplement on metabolic mediators in patients with pancreatic cancer cachexia', *Nutrition and cancer*, 40: 118-124.

Barham, J.B., M.B. Edens, A.N. Fonteh, M.M. Johnson, L. Easter and F. H. Chilton (2000), 'Addition of eicosapentaenoic acid to gamma-linolenic acid-supplemented diets prevents serum arachidonic acid accumulation in humans', *Journal of nutrition*, 130: 1925-1931.

Barkow, J., L. Cosmides and J. Tooby (eds.) (1992), *The adapted mind: evolutionary psychology and the generation of culture.* Oxford: Oxford University Press.

Baron, J.H., and A. Sonnenberg (2001), 'Period- and cohort-age contours of deaths from gastric and duodenal ulcer in New York 1804-1998', *American journal of gastroenterology*, 96: 2887-2891.

Baron, J.H., and A. Sonnenberg (2002), 'Hospital admissions for peptic ulcer and indigestion in London and New York in the 19th and early 20th centuries', *Gut*, 50: 568-570.

Bashir, S.A. (2002), 'Home is where the harm is: inadequate housing as a public health crisis', *American journal of public health*, 92: 733-738.

Baxter, L.R., J.M. Schwartz, K.S. Bergman, M.P. Szuba, B.H. Guze, J.C. Mazziotta, A. Akazraju, C.E. Selin, H.K. Ferng, P. Munford and M.E. Phelps (1992), 'Caudate glucose metabolic rate changes with both drug and behavior therapy for obsessive-compulsive disorder', *Archives of general psychiatry*, 49: 681-689.

Bechtel, W. (1988), *Philosophy of mind: an overview for cognitive science.* Hillsdale, New Jersey: Erlbaum.

Bechtel, W., and A. Abrahamsen (1991), *Connectionism and the mind: an introduction to parallel processing in networks.* Oxford: Blackwell.

Bechtel, W., and R.C. Richardson (1993), *Discovering complexity: decomposition and localization strategies in scientific research.* Princeton: Princeton University Press.

Bekelman, J.E., Y. Li and C.P. Gross (2003), 'Scope and impact of financial conflicts of interest in biomedical research: a systematic review', *Journal of the American Medical Association*, 289: 454-465.

Bender, D.A. (2002), *Introduction to nutrition and metabolism*, 3rd ed. London: Taylor & Francis.

Bennett, R.M. (ed.) (2002), *The clinical neurobiology of fibromyalgia and myofascial pain: therapeutic implications.* New York: Haworth Medical Press.

Bensoussan, A., N.J. Talley, M. Hing, R. Menzies, A. Guo and M. Ngu (2000), 'Treatment of irritable bowel syndrome with Chinese herbal medicine', in: P.B. Fontanarosa (ed.), *Alternative medicine: an objective assessment.* American Medical Association, JAMA and Archives / Journals, 342-349.

Berg, C., and P. Södersten (1998), 'Anorexia nervosa: rediscovery of a disorder', *Lancet*, 351: 1427-1429.

Beutler, L.E., and M.L. Malik (2002), *Rethinking the DSM: a psychological perspective.* Washington, D.C.: American Psychological Association.

Binder, E.B., B. Kinkead, M.J. Owens and C.B. Nemeroff (2001), 'The role of neurotensin in the pathophysiology of schizophrenia and the mechanism of action of antipsychotic drugs', *Biological psychiatry*, 50: 856-872.

Bingham, C.O. 3rd (2002), 'Development and clinical application of COX-2-selective inhibitors for the treatment of osteoarthritis and rheumatoid arthritis', *Cleveland Clinic journal of medicine*, 69, Supplement 1: SI5-S12.

Birch, S. (1998), 'Diversity and acupuncture: acupuncture is not a coherent or historically stable tradition', in: A. Vickers (ed.), *Examining complementary medicine.* Cheltenham: Stanley Thornes, 45-63.

Blackmore, S. (1993), *Dying to live: science and the near-death experience.* London: HarperCollins Publishers.

Block, N., O. Flanagan and G. Güzeldere (1997), *The nature of consciousness: philosophical debates.* Cambridge, Massachusetts: MIT Press.

Blumberg, M.S. (2002), *Body heat: temperature and life on earth.* Cambridge, Massachusetts: Harvard University Press.

Bodeker, G., and M.L. Willcox (2000), 'The first international meeting of the Research Initiative on Traditional Antimalarial Methods (RITAM)', *Journal of alternative and complementary medicine*, 6: 195-207.

Bolton, D., and J. Hill (1996), *Mind, meaning and mental disorder.* Oxford: Oxford University Press.

Bootzin, R.R., and O. Caspi (2002), 'Explanatory mechanisms for placebo effects: cognition, personality and social learning', in: H.A. Guess, A. Kleinman, J.W. Kusek and L.W. Engel (eds.), *The science of the placebo: toward an interdisciplinary research agenda.* London: BMJ Books, 108-131.

Boseley, S. (2003), 'WHO 'infiltrated by food industry'', *Guardian,* 9 January.

Boska, M.D., K.M. Welch, P.B. Barker, J.A. Nelson and L. Schultz

(2002), 'Contrasts in cortical magnesium, phospholipid and energy metabolism between migraine syndromes', *Neurology*, 58: 1227-1233.

Bowers, L. (1998), *The social nature of mental illness.* London: Routledge.

Boyle, M. (2002), *Schizophrenia: a scientific delusion?,* 2nd ed. Hove, East Sussex: Routledge.

Brady, E. (ed.) (2001), *Healing logics: culture and medicine in modern health belief systems.* Logan, Utah: Utah State University Press.

Brandon, R.N. (1990), *Adaptation and environment.* Princeton: Princeton University Press.

Brody, H., and D. Brody (1997), *The placebo response: how you can release the body's inner pharmacy for better health*. New York: HarperCollins Publishers.

Brooke, M.H. (2001), 'The classification of muscle diseases', in: G. Karpati, D. Hilton-Jones and R.C. Griggs (eds.), *Disorders of voluntary muscle*, 7th ed. Cambridge: Cambridge University Press, 374-384.

Bucher, H.C., P. Hengstler, C. Schindler and G. Meier (2002), 'N-3 polyunsaturated fatty acids in coronary heart disease: a meta-analysis of randomized controlled trials', *American journal of medicine*, 112: 298-304.

Buckley, M.J., and C.A. O'Morain (1998), '*Helicobacter* biology – discovery', *British medical bulletin*, 54: 7-16.

Buller, D.J. (ed.) (1999), *Function, selection and design.* Albany: State University of New York Press.

Burdon, R.H. (1999), *Genes and the environment.* London: Taylor & Francis.

Burian, R., R.C. Richardson and W.J. van der Steen (1996), 'Against generality: meaning and reference in genetics and philosophy', *Studies in history and philosophy of science*, 27: 1-29.

Burns, M.J. (2001), 'The pharmacology and toxicology of atypical antipsychotic agents', *Journal of toxicology and clinical toxicology*, 39: 1-14.

Buschmann, J., G. Leppla-Wollsiffer, N. Nemeth, K. Nelson and R. Kirsten (1996), 'Migraine patients show increased platelet vasopressin receptors', *Headache*, 36: 586-588.

Buss, D.M. (1995), 'Evolutionary psychology: a new paradigm for social science', *Psychological inquiry*, 6: 1-30.

Cady, R.K. (1999), 'Diagnosis and treatment of migraine', *Clinical cornerstone*, 1: 21-32.

Calder, P.C. (1997), 'N-3 polyunsaturated fatty acids and cytokine production in health and disease', *Annals of nutrition & metabolism*, 41: 203-234.

Calder, P.C. (2002), 'Dietary modification of inflammation with lipids', *Proceedings of the Nutritional Society*, 61: 345-358.

Calder, P.C., and R.B. Zurier (2001), 'Polyunsaturated fatty acids and rheumatoid arthritis', *Current opinion in clinical nutrition and metabolic care*, 4: 115-121.

Calder, P.C., and R.F. Grimble (2002), 'Polyunsaturated fatty acids, inflammation and immunity', *European journal of clinical nutrition*, 56, Supplement 3: S14-S19.

Campbell, D.R., M.M. Haber, E. Sheldon, C. Collis, N. Lukasik, B. Huang and J.L. Goldstein (2002), 'Effect of H. pylori status on gastric ulcer healing in patients continuing nonsteroidal anti-inflammatory therapy and receiving treatment with lansoprazole or ranitidine', *American journal of gastroenterology*, 97: 2208-2214.

Campling, F., and M. Sharpe (2000), *Chronic fatigue syndrome (CFS/ME): the facts.* Oxford: Oxford University Press.

Caplan, P.J. (1995), *They say you're crazy: how the world's most powerful psychiatrists decide who's normal.* Reading, Massachusetts: Addison-Wesley.

Carmody, D., and J.T. Carmody (1996), *Mysticism: holiness East and*

West. New York: Oxford University Press.

Carson, R.C. (1997), 'Costly compromises: a critique of the diagnostic and statistical manual of mental disorders', in: S. Fisher and R.P. Greenberg (eds.), *From placebo to panacea: putting psychiatric drugs to the test.* New York: John Wiley & Sons, 98-112.

Carter, R., and K.N. Mendis (2002), 'Evolutionary and historical aspects of the burden of malaria', *Clinical microbiology reviews*, 15: 564-594.

Caudill, E. (1997), *Darwinian myths: the legends and misuses of a theory.* Knoxville: University of Tennessee Press.

Cavalli-Sforza, L.L. (2000), *Genes, peoples, and languages.* Berkeley: University of California Press.

Chalmers, A., G.O. Littlejohn, I. Salit and F. Wolfe (eds.) (1995), *Fibromyalgia, chronic fatigue syndrome, and repetitive strain injury.* New York: Haworth Medical Press.

Charles, D. (2001), *Lords of the harvest: biotech, big money, and the future of food.* Cambridge, Massachusetts: Perseus Publishing.

Chibmall, J.T., J.M. Jeral and M.A. Cerullo (2001), 'Experiments on distant intercessory prayer: God, science, and the lesson of Massah', *Archives of internal medicine*, 161: 2529-2536.

Chikanza, I.C., and A.S. Grossman (1998), 'Hypothalamic-pituitary-mediated immunomodulation: arginine vasopressin is a neuroendocrine immune mediator', *British journal of rheumatology*, 37: 131-136.

Childs, B. (1999), *Genetic medicine: a logic of disease.* Baltimore: Johns Hopkins University Press.

Chivian, E., M. McCally, H. Hu and A. Haines (1993), *Critical condition: human health and the environment.* Cambridge, Massachusetts: MIT Press.

Christensen, J.H., and E.B. Schmidt (2001), 'N-3 fatty acids and the risk of sudden cardiac death', *Lipids*, 36, Supplement: S115-S118.

Christensen, P.B., K.E. Albertsen and P. Jensen (1993), 'Renal failure after omeprazole', *Lancet*, 341: 55.

Churchland, P.S. (2002), *Brain-wise: studies in neurophilosophy.* Cambridge, Massachusetts: MIT Press.

Clandinin, M.T., and J. Jumpsen (1997), 'Fatty acid metabolism in brain in relation to development, membrane structure, and signaling', in: S. Yehuda and D.I. Mostofsky (eds.), *Handbook of essential fatty acid biology: biochemistry, physiology, and behavioral neurobiology.* Totowa, New Jersey: Humana Press, 15-65.

Clark, A. (1997), *Being there: putting brain, body, and world together again.* Cambridge, Massachusetts: MIT Press.

Cleland, L.G., C.L. Hill and M.J. James (1995), 'Diet and arthritis', *Baillieres clinical rheumatology*, 9: 771-785.

Cohen, D. (1997), 'A critique of the use of neuroleptic drugs in psychiatry', in: S. Fisher and R.P. Greenberg (eds.), *From placebo to panacea: putting psychiatric drugs to the test.* New York: John Wiley & Sons, 173-228.

Constantinescu, C.S. (2002), 'Migraine and Raynaud phenomenon: possible late complications of Kawasaki disease', *Headache*, 42: 227-229.

Coppock, V., and J. Hopton (2000), *Critical perspectives on mental health.* London: Routledge.

Cosmides, L., and J. Tooby (1994), 'Beyond intuition and instinct blindness: toward an evolutionary rigorous cognitive science', *Cognition*, 50: 41-77.

Coste, J., C. Hanotin and E. Leutenegger (1995), 'Prescription of non-steroidal anti-inflammatory agents and risk of iatrogenic adverse effects: a survey of 1072 French general practitioners' [French], *Therapie*, 50: 265-270.

Covelli, V., A.B. Maffione, C. Nacci, E. Tato and E. Jirillo (1998), 'Stress, neuropsychiatric disorders and immunological effects exerted by benzodiazepines', *Immunopharmacology and immunotoxicology*, 20: 199-209.

Cox, N.H. (1992), 'Acute disseminated epidermal necrosis due to omeprazole', *Lancet*, 340: 857.

Crick, F. (1994), *The astonishing hypothesis: the scientific search for the soul.* London: Simon & Schuster.

Cunningham, A.J. (2002), 'A new approach to testing the effects of group psychological therapy on length of life in patients with metastatic cancers', *Advances in mind-body medicine*, 18: 5-9.

Danton, W.G., and D.O. Antonuccio (1997), 'A focused empirical analysis of treatments for panic and anxiety', in: S. Fisher and R.P. Greenberg (eds.), *From placebo to panacea: putting psychiatric drugs to the test.* New York: John Wiley & Sons, 229-280.

Das, U.N. (1998), 'Hypothesis: cis-unsaturated fatty acids as potential anti-peptic ulcer drugs', *Prostaglandins, leukotrienes, and essential fatty acids*, 58: 377-380.

Davidoff, R.A. (2002), *Migraine: manifestations, pathogenesis, and management,* 2nd ed. New York: Oxford University Press.

Davies, P.S. (1996), 'Discovering the functional mesh: on the methods of evolutionary psychology', *Minds and machines*, 6: 559-585.

Dawes, R.M. (1994), *House of cards: psychology and psychotherapy built on myth.* New York: The Free Press.

De Boer, W.A., and G.N.J. Tytgat (2000), 'Treatment of *Helicobacter pylori* infection', *British medical journal*, 320: 31-34.

Defromont L., C. Portenart and A. Couvez (1999), 'Psychiatric side effects of non-steroidal anti-inflammatory agents' [French], *Encephale*, 25: 11-15.

Deharo, E., G. Bourdy, C. Quenevo, V. Munoz, G. Ruiz and M. Sauvain (2001), 'A search for natural bioactive compounds in Bolivia through a multidisciplinary approach. Part V. Evaluation of the antimalarial activity of plants used by the Tacana Indians', *Journal of ethnopharmacology*, 77: 91-98.

DeLuca, P., D. Rothman and R.B. Zurier (1995), 'Marine and botanical lipids as immunomodulatory and therapeutic agents in the treatment of rheumatoid arthritis', *Rheumatic diseases in the clinics of North America*, 21: 759-777.

De Tommaso, M., D. Murasecco, G. Libro, M. Guido, V. Sciruicchio, L.M. Specchio, V. Gallai and F. Puca (2002), 'Modulation of trigeminal reflex excitability in migraine: effects of attention and habituation on the blink reflex', *International journal of psychophysiology*, 44: 239-249.

Diamond, S., and R. Wenzel (2002), 'Practical approaches to migraine management', *CNS drugs*, 16: 385-340.

Dienstfrey, H. (2000), 'Tabulating the results', *Advances in mind-body medicine*, 16: 28-32.

Djulbegovic, B., M. Lacevic, A. Cantor, K.K. Fields, C.L. Bennett, J.R. Adams, N.M. Kuderer and G.H. Lyman (2000), 'The uncertainty principle and industry-sponsored research', *Lancet*, 356: 635-638.

Dominici, P., S. Bellentani, A.R. Di Biase, G. Saccoccio, A. Le Rose, F. Masutti, L. Viola, F. Balli, C. Tiribelli, R. Grilli, M. Fusillo and E. Grossi (1999), 'Familial clustering of *Helicobacter pylori* infection: population based study', *British medical journal*, 319: 537-541.

Double, D. (2002), 'The limits of psychiatry', *British medical journal*, 324: 900-904.

Drago, L., B. Mombelli, G. Ciardo, E. De Vecchi and M.R. Gismondo (1999), 'Effects of three different fish oil formulations on *Helicobacter pylori* growth and viability: in vitro study', *Journal of chemotherapy*, 11: 207-210.

Dreier, J.P., J. Kleeberg, G. Petzold, J. Priller, O. Windmuller, H.D. Orzechowski, U. Lindauer, U. Heinemann, K.M. Einhaupl and U. Dirnagl (2002), 'Endothelin-1 potently induces Leao's cortical spreading depression in vivo in the rat: a model for an endothelial trigger of migrainous aura?', *Brain*, 125: 102-112.

Dugatkin, L.L. (2000), *The imitation factor: evolution beyond the gene.* New York: The Free Press.

Duncan, B. (2001), *CFIDS, fibromyalgia, and the virus-allergy link.* New

York: Haworth Medical Press.

Dunford, C., R. Cooper, P. Molan and R. White (2000), 'The use of honey in wound management', *Nursing standard*, 15: 63-68.

Dye, C., and M.A. Espinal (2001), 'Will tuberculosis become resistant to all antibiotics?', *Proceedings of the Royal Society London, B, biological sciences*, 268: 45-52.

Eaton, S.B., and M. Konner (1985), 'Paleolithic nutrition: a consideration of its nature and current implications', *New England journal of medicine*, 312: 283-289.

Ebneter, M., M. Binder and R. Saller (2001), 'Fernheilung und klinische Forschung', *Forschende Komplementärmedizin und klassische Naturheilkunde*, 8: 274-287.

Edwards, R., M. Peet, J. Shay and D. Horrobin (1998), 'Omega-3 polyunsaturated fatty acid levels in the diet and in red blood cell membranes of depressed patients', *Journal of affective disorders*, 48: 149-155.

Elman, J.L., E.A. Bates, M.H. Johnson, A. Karmiloff-Smith, D. Parisi and K. Plunkett (1996), *Rethinking innateness: a connectionist perspective on development.* Cambridge, Massachusetts: MIT Press.

Elmstahl, S., U. Svensson and G. Berglund (1998), 'Fermented milk products are associated to ulcer disease. Results from a cross-sectional population study', *European journal of clinical nutrition*, 52: 668-674.

Empl, M., P. Sostak, M. Breckner, M. Riedel, N. Muller, R. Gruber, S. Forderreuther and A. Straube (1999), 'T-cell subsets and expression of integrins in peripheral blood of patients with migraine', *Cephalalgia*, 19: 713-717.

Emsley, R., C. Myburgh, P. Oosthuizen and S.J. van Rensburg (2002), 'Randomized, placebo-controlled study of ethyl-eicosapentaenoic acid as supplemental treatment in schizophrenia', *American journal of psychiatry*, 159: 1596-1598.

Engel, G.L. (1977), 'The need for a new medical model: a challenge for biomedicine', *Science*, 196: 129-136.

Engel, G.L. (1981), 'The clinical application of the biopsychosocial model', *Journal of medicine and philosophy*, 6: 101-123.

Engler, M.B., M.M. Engler, A. Browne, Y.P. Sun and R. Sievers (2000), 'Mechanisms of vasorelaxation induced by eicosapentaenoic acid (20:5n-3) in WKY rat aorta', *British journal of pharmacology*, 131: 1793-1799.

Epstein, S.S. (1998), *The politics of cancer revisited.* New York: East Ridge Press.

Erasmus, U. (1993), *Fats that heal, fats that kill,* 2nd ed. Burnaby: Alive Books.

Ergas, D., E. Eilat, S. Mendlovic and Z.M. Sthoeger (2002), 'N-3 fatty acids and the immune system in autoimmunity', *Israel medical association journal*, 4: 34-38.

Ernst, P.B., and J. Pappo (2001), 'T-cell-mediated mucosal immunity in the absence of antibody: lessons from *Helicobacter pylori* infection', *Acta odontologica Scandinavica*, 59: 216-221.

Ernst, P.B., H. Takaishi and S.E. Crowe (2001), '*Helicobacter pylori* infection as a model for gastrointestinal immunity and chronic inflammatory diseases', *Digestive diseases*, 19: 104-111.

Eskandari, F., and E.M. Sternberg (2002), 'Neuroendocrine mediators of placebo effects on immunity', in: H.A. Guess, A. Kleinman, J.W. Kusek and L.W. Engel (eds.), *The science of the placebo: toward an interdisciplinary research agenda*. London: BMJ Books, 169-182.

Evans, D. (1993), *Spirituality and human nature.* Albany: State University of New York Press.

Even, C., E. Siobud-Dorocant and R.M. Dardennes (2000), 'Critical approach to antidepressant trials. Blindness protection is necessary, feasible and measurable', *British journal of psychiatry*, 177: 47-51.

Ewald, P.W. (1994), *Evolution of infectious diseases.* Oxford: Oxford University Press.

Fancher, R.T. (1995), *Cultures of healing: correcting the image of*

American mental health care. New York: Freeman.

Farmer, P. (1997), *Infections and inequalities: the modern plagues*, updated ed. Berkeley: University of California Press.

Farmer, P. (2001), 'DOTS and DOTS-plus: not the only answer', *Annals of the New York Academy of Science*, 953: 165-184.

Farthing, M.J., R. Fitzgerald and Z.W. Zhang (2001), 'Acid, *Helicobacter* and immunity: a new paradigm for oesophagogastric cancer', *Journal of physiology, Paris*, 95: 423-427.

Faust, T., J.S. Redfern, E. Lee and M. Feldman (1989), 'Effects of fish oil on gastric mucosal 6-keto-PGF1 alpha synthesis and ethanol-induced injury', *American journal of physiology*, 257: G9-G13.

Fava, G.A. (2002), 'Conflict of interest and the credibility of clinical medicine: a psychosomatic antidote', in: T. Sivik, D. Byrne, D. Lipsitt, G. Christodoulou and H. Dienstfrey (eds.), *Psycho-neuro-endocrino-immunology (PNEI).* Amsterdam: Elsevier, 229-236.

Fenton, W.S., F. Dickerson, J. Boronow, J.R. Hibbeln and M. Knable (2001), 'A placebo-controlled trial of omega-3 fatty acid (ethyl eicosapentaenoic acid) supplementation for residual symptoms and cognitive impairment in schizophrenia', *American journal of psychiatry*, 158: 2071-2074.

Fenwick, P. (1997), 'Is the near-death experience only N-methyl-D-aspartate blocking?', *Journal of near-death studies*, 16: 43-53.

Fischer, C.S., M. Hout, M.S. Jankowski, S.R. Lucas, A. Swidler and K. Voss (1996), *Inequality by design: cracking the bell curve myth.* Princeton, New Jersey: Princeton University Press.

Fisher, P. (1998), 'Is homeopathic prescribing reliable?', in: A. Vickers (ed.), *Examining complementary medicine.* Cheltenham: Stanley Thornes, 74-87.

Fisher, S., and R.P. Greenberg (1997), 'The curse of the placebo: fanciful pursuit of a pure biological therapy', in: S. Fisher and R.P. Greenberg (eds.), *From placebo to panacea: putting psychiatric drugs to the test.* New York: John Wiley & Sons, 3-56.

Flammer, J., M. Pache and T. Resink (2001), 'Vasospasm, its role in the pathogenesis of diseases with particular reference to the eye', *Progress in retinal eye research*, 20: 319-349.

Fontanarosa, P.B. (2000), *Alternative medicine: an objective assessment.* American Medical Association, JAMA and Archives / Journals.

Forman, R. (ed.) (1990), *The problem of pure consciousness: mysticism and philosophy.* New York: Oxford University Press.

Fox, M. (2003), *Religion, spirituality and the near-death experience.* London: Routledge.

Frank, M.G., J.L. Wieseler Frank, S.E. Hendricks, W.J. Burke and D.R. Johnson (2002), 'Age at onset of major depressive disorder predicts reductions in NK cell number and activity', *Journal of affective disorders*, 71: 159-167.

Frank, S.A. (2002), *Immunology and evolution of infectious disease.* Princeton: Princeton University Press.

Franzek, E., and H. Beckmann (1999), *Psychoses of the schizophrenic spectrum in twins.* Vienna: Springer.

Fuller, S. (2002), 'The trouble with facts: an obsession with scientific evidence is leading politicians into dangerous waters', *New scientist*, 2348: 46-47.

Garcia Rodriguez, L.A., and A. Ruigomez (1997), 'Gastric acid, acid-suppressing drugs, and bacterial gastroenteritis: how much of a risk?', *Epidemiology*, 8: 571-574.

Garfield, R. (1999), 'Malaria control in Nicaragua: social and political influences on disease transmission and control activities', *Lancet*, 354: 414-418.

Garrett, L. (1994), *The coming plague: newly emerging diseases in a world out of balance.* New York: Farrar, Straus and Giroux.

Gazzaniga, M.S. (ed.) (2000), *The new cognitive neurosciences*, 2nd ed. Cambridge, Massachusetts: MIT Press.

Geddes, J., N. Freemantle, P. Harrison and P. Bebbington (2000), 'Atypical antipsychotics in the treatment of schizophrenia: systematic overview and meta-regression analysis', *British medical journal*, 321: 1371-1376.

Gellman, J. (2001), *Mystical experience of God: a philosophical inquiry.* Aldershot: Ashgate.

Gharzouli, K., A. Gharzouli, S. Amira and S. Khennouf (2001), 'Protective effect of mannitol, glucose-fructose-sucrose-maltose mixture, and natural honey hyperosmolar solutions against ethanol-induced gastric mucosal damage in rats', *Experimental and toxicologic pathology*, 53: 175-180.

Giffin, N.J., and H. Kaube (2002), 'The electrophysiology of migraine', *Current opinions in neurology*, 15: 303-309.

Gijswijt-Hofstra, M., and R. Porter (1998). *Cultures of psychiatry.* Amsterdam: Rodopi.

Gilbert, P., and K.G. Bailey (2000), *Genes on the couch: explorations in evolutionary psychotherapy.* East-Sussex: Brunner-Routledge.

Glassman, A.H. (2002), 'Clinical management of cardiovascular risks during treatment with psychotropic drugs', *Journal of clinical psychiatry*, 63, Supplement 9: S12-S17.

Goenka, K., R. Kochhar, A. Chakrabarti, A. Kumar, O. Gupta, P. Talwar and S.K. Mehta (1996), 'Candida overgrowth after treatment of duodenal ulcer; a comparison of cimetidine, famotidine, and omeprazole', *Journal of clinical gastroenterology*, 23: 7-10.

Goetsche, P.C. (1989), 'Methodology and overt and hidden bias in reports in 196 double-blind trials of nonsteroid anti-inflammatory drugs in rheumatoid arthritis', *Controlled clinical trials*, 10: 31-56.

Goodkin, K., and A.P. Visser (2000), *Psychoneuroimmunology: stress, mental disorders and health.* Washington, D.C.: American Psychiatric Press.

Goodman, K.W. (2003), *Ethics and evidence-based medicine: fallibility and responsibility in clinical science.* Cambridge: Cambridge University Press.

Goodwin, C.S. (1994), 'How *Helicobacter pylori* acquired its name, and how it overcomes gastric defence mechanisms', *Journal of gastroenterology and hepatology*, 9, Supplement 1: S1-S3.

Goodwin, J.S., and M.R. Tangum (2000), 'Battling quackery: attitudes about micronutrient supplements', in: P.B. Fontanarosa (ed.), *Alternative medicine: an objective assessment*. American Medical Association, JAMA and Archives / Journals, 216-221.

Gordon, R.J., B.C. Nienstedt and W.M. Gesler (1998), *Alternative therapies: expanding options in health care.* New York: Springer.

Graham, D.Y. (2002), 'Critical effect of *Helicobacter pylori* infection on the effectiveness of omeprazole for prevention of gastric or duodenal ulcers among chronic NSAID users', *Helicobacter*, 7: 1-8.

Gray, D., and P. Toghill (eds.) (2001), *An introduction to the symptoms and signs of clinical medicine*. London: Arnold.

Greenberg, M.D. (1997), 'Treatment implications of psychiatric comorbidity', in: S. Fisher and R.P. Greenberg (eds.), *From placebo to panacea: putting psychiatric drugs to the test.* New York: John Wiley & Sons, 57-97.

Greenberg, R.P., and S. Fisher (1997), 'Mood-mending medicines: probing drug, psychotherapy, and placebo solutions', in: S. Fisher and R.P. Greenberg (eds.), *From placebo to panacea: putting psychiatric drugs to the test.* New York: John Wiley & Sons, 115-172.

Greyson, B. (2000), 'Near-death experiences', in: E. Cardeña, S.J. Lynn and S. Krippner (eds.), *Varieties of anomalous experience*. Washington, D.C.: American Psychological Association, 315-352.

Griffin, M.R. (1998), 'Epidemiology of nonsteroidal anti-inflammatory drug-associated gastrointestinal injury', *American journal of medicine*, 104: S23-S29, S41-S42.

Griffiths, P.E. (1996), 'The historical turn in the study of adaptation', *British journal for the philosophy of science*, 47: 511-532.

Grimble, R.F. (2001), 'Nutritional modulation of immune function', *Proceedings of the Nutrition Society*, 60: 389-397.

Grimm, H., K. Mayer, P. Mayser and E. Eigenbrodt (2002), 'Regulatory potential of n-3 fatty acids in immunological and inflammatory processes', *British journal of nutrition* 87, Supplement 1: S59-S67.

Groff, J.L., S.S. Gropper and S.M. Hunt (1995), *Advanced nutrition and human metabolism*, 2nd ed. St. Paul, Minneapolis: West Publishing Company.

Guidetti, V., F. Galli, P. Fabrizi, A.S. Giannantoni, L. Napoli, O. Bruni and S. Trillo (1998), 'Headache and psychiatric comorbidity: clinical aspects and outcome in an 8-year follow-up study', *Cephalalgia*, 18: 455-462.

Gull, W. (1874), 'Anorexia nervosa (apapsia hysterica, anorexia hysterica)', *Transactions of the Clinical Society of London*, 7: 22-28.

Gupta, V.K. (1997), 'A clinical review of the adaptive role of vasopressin in migraine', *Cephalalgia*, 17: 561-569.

Guthrie, S.E. (1993), *Faces in the clouds: a new theory of religion.* New York: Oxford University Press.

Guzel, C., G. Ulak, A. Sermet, R. Cicek and M. Ulak (1995), 'Effect of fish oil on indometacin-induced gastric lesions in rats', *Arzneimittelforschung*, 45: 1172-1173.

Hanington, E., R.J. Jones, J.A. Amess and B. Wachowicz (1981), 'Migraine: a platelet disorder', *Lancet*, 2: 720-723.

al-Harbi, M.M., M.W. Islam, O.A. al-Shabanah and N.M. al-Gharably (1995), 'Effect of acute administration of fish oil (omega-3 marine triglyceride) on gastric ulceration and secretion induced by various ulcerogenic and necrotizing agents in rats', *Food chemical toxicology*, 33: 553-558.

Hardwicke, C.J. (2002), 'The World Health Organization and the pharmaceutical industry: common areas of interest and differing views', *Adverse drug reactions and toxicology reviews*, 21: 51-99.

Harel, Z., G. Gascon, S. Riggs, R. Vaz, W. Brown and G. Exil (2002), 'Supplementation with omega-3 polyunsaturated fatty acids in the management of recurrent migraines in adolescents', *Journal of adolescent health*, 31: 54-61.

Harper, C.R., and T.A. Jacobson (2001), 'The fats of life: the role of omega-3 fatty acids in the prevention of coronary heart disease', *Archives of internal medicine*, 161: 2185-2192.

Harrington, A. (ed.) (1997), *The placebo effect: an interdisciplinary exploration.* Cambridge, Massachusetts: Harvard University Press.

Harrington, A. (2002), '"Seeing" the placebo effect: historical legacies and present opportunities', in: H.A. Guess, A. Kleinman, J.W. Kusek and L.W. Engel (eds.), *The science of the placebo: toward an interdisciplinary research agenda.* London: BMJ Books, 35-52.

Hartl, D.L., S.K. Volkman, K.M. Nielsen, A.E. Barry, K.P. Day, D.F. Wirth and E.A. Winzeler (2002), 'The paradoxical population genetics of *Plasmodium falciparum*', *Trends in parasitology*, 18: 266-272.

Hasselblatt, M., J. Kohler, E. Volles and H. Ehrenreich (1999), 'Simultaneous monitoring of endothelin-1 and vasopressin plasma levels in migraine', *Neuroreport*, 10: 423-425.

Hawkey, C.J. (2002), 'Cyclooxygenase inhibition: between the devil and the deep blue sea', *Gut*, 50, Supplement 3: S25-S30.

Healy, D. (2002), *The creation of psychopharmacology.* Cambridge, Massachusetts: Harvard University Press.

Heinrichs, R.W. (2001), *In search of madness: schizophrenia and neuroscience.* Oxford: Oxford University Press.

Hellstrom, H.R. (1999), 'The altered homeostatic theory: a holistic approach to multiple diseases, including atherosclerosis, ischemic diseases, and hypertension', *Medical hypotheses*, 53: 194-199.

Helzer, J.E., and J.J. Hudziak (eds.) (2002), *Defining psychopathology in the 21st century: DSM-V and beyond.* Washington, D.C.: American Psychopathological Association.

Herrnstein, R.J., and C. Murray (1994), *The bell curve: intelligence and class structure in American life.* New York: The Free Press.

Hess, D.J. (1999), *Evaluating alternative cancer therapies: a guide to the science and politics of an emerging medical field.* New Brunswick, New Jersey and London: Rutgers University Press.

Ho, M.-W. (1998), *Genetic engineering: dream or nightmare?* Dublin: Gateway.

Hobohm, U. (2001), 'Fever and cancer in perspective', *Cancer immunology and immunotherapy*, 50: 391-396.

Hoffer, A. (1998), *Vitamin B-3, schizophrenia: discovery, recovery, controversy.* Kingston, Ontario: Quarry Press.

Holman, R.T. (1997), 'Omega3 and omega6 essential fatty acid status in human health and disease', in: S. Yehuda and D.I. Mostofsky (eds.), *Handbook of essential fatty acid biology: biochemistry, physiology, and behavioral neurobiology.* Totowa, New Jersey: Humana Press, 139-182.

Hoption Cann, S.A., J.P. van Netten, C. van Netten and D.W. Glover (2002), 'Spontaneous regression: a hidden treasure buried in time', *Medical hypotheses*, 58: 115-119.

Horrobin, D.F. (1997), 'Fatty acids, phospholipids, and schizophrenia', in: S. Yehuda and D.I. Mostofsky (eds.), *Handbook of essential fatty acid biology: biochemistry, physiology, and behavioral neurobiology.* Totowa, New Jersey: Humana Press, 245-256.

Horrobin, D.F. (2000), 'Commentary on the workshop statement: are we really sure that arachidonic acid and linoleic acid are bad things?', *Prostaglandins, leukotrienes, and essential fatty acids*, 63: 145-147.

Horrobin, D.F. (2001), 'Phospholipid metabolism and depression: the possible roles of phospholipase A2 and coenzyme A-independent transacylase', *Human psychopharmacology*, 16: 45-52.

Horrobin, D.F. (2002), 'A new category of psychotropic drugs: neuroactive lipids as exemplified by ethyl eicosapentaenoate (E-E)', *Progress in drug research*, 59: 171-199.

Horrobin, D.F., K. Jenkins, C.N. Bennett and W.W. Christie (2002), 'Eicosapentaenoic acid and arachidonic acid: collaboration and not antagonism is the key to biological understanding', *Prostaglandins, leukotrienes, and essential fatty acids*, 66: 83-90.

Horton, R. (2002), 'WHO: the casualties and compromises of renewal', *Lancet*, 359: 1605-1611.

Howe, M.J.A. (1997), *IQ in question: the truth about intelligence.* London: Sage Publications.

Hu, F.B., L. Bronner, W.C. Willett, M.J. Stampfer, K.M. Rexrode, C.M. Albert, D. Hunter and J.E. Manson (2002), 'Fish and omega-3 fatty acid intake and risk of coronary heart disease in women', *Journal of the American Medical Association*, 287: 1815-1821.

Hughes, D.A., and A.C. Pinder (2000), 'N-3 polyunsaturated fatty acids inhibit the antigen-presenting function of human monocytes', *American journal of clinical nutrition*, 71: S357-S360.

Humber, J.M., and R.F. Almeder (eds.) (1997), *What is disease?* Totowa, New Jersey: Humana Press.

IMS Health Canada (1999), 'New arthritis medication achieves fastest adoption ever recorded in Canada', *Newsletter September*.

Innocenti, M., A.C. Thoreson, R.L. Ferrero, E. Stromberg, I. Bolin, L. Eriksson, A.M. Svennerholm and M. Quiding-Jarbrink (2002), '*Helicobacter pylori*-induced activation of human endothelial cells', *Infection and immunity*, 70: 4581-4590.

Itzkoff, S.W. (1994), *The decline of intelligence in America.* Westport: Praeger.

Jacobs, D.H. (1995), 'Psychiatric drugging: forty years of pseudo-science, self-interest, and indifference to harm', *The journal of mind and behavior*, 16: 421-470.

Jacobs, D.H. (1999), 'A close and critical examination of how psychopharmacotherapy research is conducted', *The journal of mind and behavior*, 20: 311-350.

Jain, A., S. Buddhiraja, B. Khurana, R. Singhal, D. Nair, P. Arora, P. Gangwal, S.K. Mishra, B. Uppal, R. Gondal and P. Kar (1999), 'Risk factors for duodenal ulcer in north India', *Tropical gastroenterology*, 20: 36-39.

James, M.J., and L.G. Cleland (1997), 'Dietary n-3 fatty acids and therapy for rheumatoid arthritis', *Seminars in arthritis and rheumatism*, 27: 85-97.

James, M.J., R.A. Gibson and L.G. Cleland (2000), 'Dietary polyunsaturated fatty acids and inflammatory mediator production', *American journal of clinical nutrition*, 71: S343-S348.

Jamin, S.P., M. Crabos, M. Catheline, C. Martin-Chouly, A.B. Legrand and B. Saiag (1999), 'Eicosapentaenoic acid reduces thrombin-evoked release of endothelin-1 in cultured bovine endothelial cells', *Research communications in molecular pathology and pharmacology*, 105: 271-281.

Jansen, K.L.R. (1997), 'The ketamine model of the near-death experience: a central role for the N-methyl-D-aspartate receptor', *Journal of near-death studies*, 16: 5-25.

Jennekens, F.G.I., and L. Kater (1999), *Neurology of the inflammatory connective tissue diseases.* London: Saunders.

Johnson, S. (2001), 'The multifaceted and widespread pathology of magnesium deficiency', *Medical hypotheses*, 56: 163-170.

Jones, B., E. Hewson and A. Price (1994), 'Acute interstitial nephritis due to omeprazole', *Lancet*, 344: 1017-1018.

Joseph, J. (1999), 'A critique of the Finnish adoptive family study of schizophrenia', *Journal of mind and behavior*, 20: 133-154.

Joseph, J. (2001), 'Is crime in the genes? A critical review of twin and adoption studies of criminality and antisocial behavior', *Journal of mind and behavior*, 22: 179-218.

Joy, C.B., R. Mumby-Croft, and L.A. Joy (2001), 'Polyunsaturated fatty acid (fish or evening primrose oil) for schizophrenia' (Cochrane Review), *The Cochrane library*, Issue 3.

Jüni, P., A.W.S. Rutjes and P.A. Dieppe (2002), 'Are selective COX 2 inhibitors superior to traditional non steroidal anti-inflammatory drugs? Adequate analysis of the CLASS trial indicates that this may not be the case', *British medical journal*, 324: 1287-1288.

Kaplan, A.S. (2002), 'Psychological treatments for anorexia nervosa: a review of published studies and promising new directions', *Canadian journal of psychiatry*, 47: 225-226.

Kaplan, J.M. (2000), *The limits and lies of human genetic research: dangers for social policy.* New York: Routledge.

Kaptchuk, T.J. (2000), *Chinese medicine: the web that has no weaver*, revised and expanded ed. London: Rider.

Kaptchuk, T.J., and D.M. Eisenberg (1998), 'Health food or granola: its truth and consequences', in: A. Vickers (ed.), *Examining complementary medicine.* Cheltenham: Stanley Thornes, 17-28.

Katz, R., J.A. Hamilton, A.A. Spector, S.A. Moore, H.W. Moser, M.J. Noetzel and P.A. Watkins (2001), 'Brain uptake and utilization of fatty acids: recommendations for future research', *Journal of molecular neuroscience*, 16: 333-335.

Kellehear, A. (1996), *Experiences near death: beyond medicine and religion.* New York: Oxford University Press.

Kelleher, J.P., F. Centorrino, M.J. Albert and R.J. Baldessarini (2002), 'Advances in atypical antipsychotics for the treatment of schizophrenia: new formulations and new agents', *CNS drugs*, 16: 249-261.

Keller, E.F. (2002), *Making sense of life: explaining biological development with models, metaphors, and machines.* Cambridge, Massachusetts: Harvard University Press.

Kelner, M., B. Wellman, B. Pescosolido and M. Saks (eds.) (2000), *Complementary and alternative medicine: challenge and change.* Amsterdam: Harwood Academic Publishers.

Kendell, R.E. (2002), 'Five criteria for an improved taxonomy of mental disorders', in: J.E. Helzer and J.J. Hudziak (eds.), *Defining psychopathology in the 21st Century: DSM-V and beyond.* Washington, D.C.: American Psychopathological Association, 3-17.

Keys, A. (ed.) (1970), 'Coronary heart disease in seven countries', *Circulation*, 41, Supplement: 1-211.

Khan, M.M., D.R. Evans, V. Gunna, R.E. Scheffer, V.V. Parikh and S.P. Mahadik (2002), 'Reduced erythrocyte membrane essential fatty acids and increased lipid peroxides in schizophrenia at the never-medicated first-episode of psychosis and after years of treatment with antipsychotics', *Schizophrenia research*, 58: 1-10.

Kiesler, D.J. (1999), *Beyond the disease model of mental disorders.* Westport: Praeger.

Killeen, G.F., U. Fillinger, I. Kiche, L.C. Gouagnaand and B.G. Knols (2002), 'Eradication of *Anopheles gambiae* from Brazil: lessons for malaria control in Africa?', *Lancet infectious diseases*, 2: 618-627.

Kim, J. (1998), *Mind in a physical world: an essay on the mind-body problem and mental causation.* Cambridge, Massachusetts: MIT Press.

Kirsch, I. (1997), 'Specifying nonspecifics: psychological mechanisms of placebo effects', in: A. Harrington (ed.), *The placebo effect: an interdisciplinary exploration.* Cambridge, Massachusetts: Harvard University Press, 166-186.

Kirsch, I., T.J. Moore, A. Scoboria and S.S. Nicholls (2002), 'The emperor's new drugs: an analysis of antidepressant medication data submitted to the U.S. Food and Drug Administration', *Prevention and treatment*, 5: 15 July.

Kirsch, I., and G. Sapirstein (1999), 'Listening to Prozac but hearing placebo: a meta-analysis of antidepressant medication', in: I. Kirsch (ed.), *How expectancies shape experience.* Washington, D.C.: American Psychological Association, 303-320.

Kissel, J.T., and R.G. Miller (1999), 'Muscle pain and fatigue', in: A.H.V. Schapira and R.C. Griggs (eds.), *Muscle diseases, blue books in practical neurology, vol. 24.* Boston: Butterworth Heinemann.

Kjaergard, L.L., and B. Als-Nielsen (2002), 'Association between competing interests and authors' conclusions: epidemiological study of randomised clinical trials published in the BMJ', *British medical journal*, 325: 249-252.

Kleinman, A., H.A. Guess and J.S. Wilentz (2002), 'An overview', in: H.A. Guess, A. Kleinman, J.W. Kusek and L.W. Engel (eds.), *The science of the placebo: toward an interdisciplinary research agenda.* London: BMJ Books, 1-32.

Kleinmuntz, B. (1990), 'Why we still use our heads instead of formulas: toward an integrative approach', *Psychological bulletin*, 107: 296-310.

Koenig, H.G. (2001), 'Religion, spirituality, and medicine: how are they related and what does it mean?', *Mayo Clinic proceedings*, 76: 1189-1191.

Koenig, H.G., and H.J. Cohen (eds.) (2002), *The link between religion and health: psychoneuroimmunology and the faith factor.* Oxford: Oxford University Press.

Kokai, M., S. Kashiwamura, H. Okamura, K. Ohara and Y. Morita (2002), 'Plasma interleukin-18 levels in patients with psychiatric disorders', *Journal of immunotherapy*, 25, Supplement 1: S68-S71.

Konradi, C., and S. Heckers (2001), 'Antipsychotic drugs and neuroplasticity: insights into the treatment and neurobiology of schizophrenia', *Biological psychiatry*, 50: 729-742.

Konstam, M.A., and M.R. Weir (2002), 'Current perspective on the cardiovascular effects of coxibs', *Cleveland Clinic journal of medicine*, 69, Supplement 1: SI47-S152.

Konturek, P.C., S.J. Konturek, M. Czesnikiewicz, M. Plonka and W. Bielanski (2002), 'Interaction of *Helicobacter pylori* (Hp) and nonsteroidal anti-inflammatory drugs (NSAID) on gastric mucosa and risk of ulcerations', *Medical science monitor*, 8: RA197-RA209.

Koo, J., and S. Arain (2000), 'Traditional Chinese medicine for the treatment of dermatologic disorders', in: P.B. Fontanarosa (ed.), *Alternative medicine: an objective assessment*. American Medical Association, JAMA and Archives / Journals, 98-105.

Kraus, A., and L.F. Flores-Suarez (1995), 'Acute gout associated with omeprazole', *Lancet*, 345: 461-462.

Kremer, J.M. (1996), 'Effects of modulation of inflammatory and immune parameters in patients with rheumatic and inflammatory disease receiving dietary supplementation of n-3 and n-6 fatty acids', *Lipids*, 31: S243-S247.

Kremer, J.M. (2000), 'N-3 fatty acid supplements in rheumatoid arthritis', *American journal of clinical nutrition*, 71: S349-S351.

Kresiun, V.I., V.M. Iurlov, A.V. Tishchenko and N.N. Oleinik (1993), 'The stress-protective effect of a new derivative of n-3-polyunsaturated fatty acids' [Russian], *Biulleten eksperimentalnoi biologii i meditsiny*, 116: 274-277.

Kristensen, S.D., A.M. Iversen and E.B. Schmidt (2001), 'N-3 polyunsaturated fatty acids and coronary thrombosis', *Lipids*, 36, Supplement: S79-S82.

Kumar, N.P., G. Wild, K.A. Ramasamy and J. Snape (2002), 'Fatal haemorrhagic pulmonary oedema and associated angioedema after the ingestion of rofecoxib', *Postgraduate medical journal*, 78: 439-440.

Kutchins, H., and S.A. Kirk (1997), *Making us crazy: DSM—the psychiatric bible and the creation of mental disorders.* New York: The Free Press.

Lacy, B.E., and J. Rosemore (2001), '*Helicobacter pylori*: ulcers and more: the beginning of an era', *Journal of nutrition*, 131: S2789-S2793.

Lagercrantz, H., M. Hanson, P. Evrard and C. Rodeck (2002), *The newborn brain: neuroscience and clinical applications.* Cambridge: Cambridge University Press.

Lake, A.E. (2001), 'Behavioral and nonpharmacologic treatments of headache', *Medical clinics of North America*, 85: 1055-1075.

Lam, S.K. (1993), 'Epidemiology and genetics of peptic ulcer', *Gastroenterologia Japanica*, 28, Supplement 5: S145-S157.

Lanas, A. (2002), 'Clinical experience with cyclooxygenase-2 inhibitors', *Rheumatology*, 41, Supplement 1: S16-S22; discussion S35-S42.

Lappé, M., and B. Bailey (1999), *Against the grain: the genetic transformation of global agriculture.* London: Earthscan.

Laugharne, J.D., J.E. Mellor and M. Peet (1996), 'Fatty acids and schizophrenia', *Lipids*, 31, Supplement: S163-S165.

Leaf, A. (2001), 'The electrophysiologic basis for the antiarrhythmic and anticonvulsant effects of n-3 polyunsaturated fatty acids: heart and brain', *Lipids*, 36, Supplement: S107-S110.

Leape, L.L. (1999), 'Error in medicine', in: M.M. Rosenthal, L. Mulcahy and S. Lloyd-Bostock (eds.), *Medical mishaps: pieces of the puzzle.* Buckingham: Open University Press, 20-38.

Leboyer, M., and F. Bellevier (eds.) (2003), *Psychiatric genetics: methods and reviews.* Totowa, New Jersey: Humana press.

LeDoux, J. (2002), *Synaptic self: how brains become how we are.* New York: Penguin.

Lema, M.J. (2002), 'Emerging options with coxib therapy', *Cleveland Clinic journal of medicine*, 69, Supplement 1: S76-S84.

Leonard, B.E., and K. Miller (eds.) (1995), *Stress, the immune system and psychiatry.* New York: John Wiley & Sons.

Lewis, C.A. (2001), 'Cultural stereotype of the effects of religion on mental health', *British journal of medical psychology*, 74: 359-367.

Lewis, C.E., R.M. O'Brien and J. Barraclough (2002), *The psychoimmunology of cancer*, 2nd, revised ed. Oxford: Oxford University Press.

Lishman, W.A. (1997), *Organic psychiatry*, revised ed. Oxford: Blackwell.

Llorca, P.M., I. Chereau, F.J. Bayle and C. Lancon (2002), 'Tardive dyskinesias and antipsychotics: a review', *European psychiatry*, 17: 129-138.

Lloyd, E.A. (1999), 'Evolutionary psychology: the burdens of proof',

Biology and philosophy, 14: 211-233.

Lohoff, M., M. Rollinghoff and F. Sommer (2000), '*Helicobacter pylori* gastritis: a Th1 mediated disease?', *Journal of biotechnology*, 83: 33-36.

Looren de Jong, H., and W.J. van der Steen (1998), 'Biological thinking in evolutionary psychology: rockbottom or quicksand?', *Philosophical psychology*, 11: 183-205.

Mackintosh, N.J. (1998), *IQ and human intelligence.* Oxford: Oxford University Press.

Madjar, I., and J.A. Walton (2001), 'What is problematic about evidence?', in: J.M. Morse, J.M. Swanson and A.J. Kuzel (eds.), *The nature of qualitative evidence.* Thousand Oaks: Sage Publications, 28-45.

Mahadik, S.P., D. Evans and H. Lal (2001), 'Oxidative stress and role of antioxidant and omega-3 essential fatty acid supplementation in schizophrenia', *Progress in Neuropsychopharmacology and biological psychiatry*, 25: 463-493.

Mandler, G. (2001), 'Apart from genetics: what makes monozygotic twins similar?', *Journal of mind and behavior*, 22: 147-159.

Mantzioris, E., L.G. Cleland, R.A. Gibson, M.A. Neumann, M. Demasi and M.J. James (2000), 'Biochemical effects of a diet containing foods enriched with n-3 fatty acids', *American journal of clinical nutrition*, 72: 42-48.

Marshall, S.J., P.F. Russell, J.D. Phillipson, G.C. Kirby, D.C. Warhurst and C.W. Wright (2000), 'Antiplasmodial and antiamoebic activities of medicinal plants from Sierra Leone', *Phytotherapy research*, 14: 356-358.

Martelletti, P., J. Sutherland, E. Anastasi, U. Di Mario and M. Giacovazzo (1989), 'Evidence for an immune-mediated mechanism in food-induced migraine from a study on activated T-cells, IgG4 subclass, anti-IgG antibodies and circulating immune complexes', *Headache*, 29: 664-670.

Martin, P. (1997), *The healing mind: the vital links between brain and behavior, immunity and disease.* New York: St. Martin's Press.

Mauskop, A., B.T. Altura and B.M. Altura (2002), 'Serum ionized magnesium levels and serum ionized calcium/ionized magnesium ratios in women with menstrual migraine', *Headache*, 42: 242-248.

Mayer, K., M. Merfels, M. Muhly-Reinholz, S. Gokorsch, S. Rosseau, J. Lohmeyer, N. Schwarzer, M. Krull, N. Suttorp, F. Grimminger and W. Seeger (2002), 'Omega-3 fatty acids suppress monocyte adhesion to human endothelial cells: role of endothelial PAF generation', *American journal of physiology, heart and circulatory physiology*, 283: H811-H818.

McClintock, A. (1995), *The convergence of machine and human nature.* Aldershot: Avebury.

McCloy, R.F., R. Arnold, K.D. Bardhan, D. Cattan, E. Klinkenberg-Knol, P.N. Maton, R.H. Riddell, P. Sipponen and A. Walan (1995), 'Pathophysiological effects of long-term acid suppression in man', *Digestive diseases and sciences*, 40: S96-S120.

McGrath, P.J. (1999), 'Clinical psychology issues in migraine headaches', *Canadian journal of neurological science*, 26, Supplement 3: S33-S36.

McGuffin, P., M.J. Owen and I.I. Gottesman (eds.) (2002), *Psychiatric genetics & genomics.* Oxford: Oxford University Press.

McGuire, M., and A. Troisi (1998), *Darwinian psychiatry.* Oxford: Oxford University Press.

McMichael, A.J. (2000), 'The urban environment and health in a world of increasing globalization: issues for developing countries', *Bulletin of the World Health Organization*, 78: 1117-1126.

Mellor, J.E., J.D. Laugharne and M. Peet (1995), 'Schizophrenic symptoms and dietary intake of n-3 fatty acids', *Schizophrenia research*, 18: 85-86.

Meltzer, H.Y., M. Davidson, A.H. Glassman and W.V. Vieweg (2002), 'Assessing cardiovascular risks versus clinical benefits of atypical antipsychotic drug treatment', *Journal of clinical psychiatry*, 63, Supplement 9: S25-S29.

Mengle-Gaw, L.J., and B.D. Schwartz (2002), 'Cyclooxygenase-2 inhibitors: promise or peril?', *Mediators of inflammation*, 11: 275-286.

Merrell, W.C., and E. Shalts (2002), 'Homeopathy', *Medical clinics of North America*, 86: 47-62.

Meurer, L.N., and D.J. Bower (2002), 'Management of *Helicobacter pylori* infection', *American family physician*, 65: 1327-1336.

Mezei, Z., B. Kis, A. Gecse, J. Tajti, B. Boda, G. Telegdy and L. Vecsei (2000), 'Platelet arachidonate cascade of migraineurs in the interictal phase', *Platelets*, 11: 222-225.

Misciagna, G., A.M. Cisternino and J. Freudenheim (2000), 'Diet and duodenal ulcer', *Digestive liver disease*, 32: 468-472.

Mitnick, C., J. Bayona, E. Palacios, S. Shin, J. Furin, F. Alcantara, E. Sanchez, M. Sarria, M. Becerra, M.C. Fawzi, S. Kapiga, D. Neuberg, J.H. Maguire, J.Y. Kim and P. Farmer (2003), 'Community-based therapy for multidrug-resistant tuberculosis in Lima, Peru', *New England journal of medicine*, 348: 119-128.

Moberg, G.P., and J.A. Mench (eds.) (2000), *The biology of animal stress: basic principles and implications for animal welfare.* New York: CAB Publishing.

Moerman, D.E. (2002), 'Explanatory mechanisms for placebo effects: cultural influences and the meaning response', in: H.A. Guess, A. Kleinman, J.W. Kusek and L.W. Engel (eds.), *The science of the placebo: toward an interdisciplinary research agenda.* London: BMJ Books, 77-107.

Moerman, D.E., and W.B. Jonas (2000), 'Toward a research agenda on placebo', with commentaries, *Advances in mind-body medicine*, 16: 3346.

Moncrieff, J. (2001), 'Are antidepressants overrated? A review of methodological problems in antidepressant trials', *Journal of nervous and mental diseases*, 189: 288-295.

Montague, P. (2000), 'Foreword', in: M. O'Brien, *Making better environmental decisions: an alternative to risk assessment.* Cambridge, Massachusetts: MIT Press, vii-x.

Moore, R.A. (2002), 'The hidden costs of arthritis treatment and the cost of new therapy – the burden of non-steroidal anti-inflammatory drug gastropathy', *Rheumatology*, 41, Supplement 1: S7-S15; discussion S35-S42.

Morris, D.B. (1997), 'Placebo, pain, and belief: a biocultural model', in: A. Harrington (ed.), *The placebo effect: an interdisciplinary exploration.* Cambridge, Massachusetts: Harvard University Press, 187-207.

Morrison, G., and L. Hark (1999), *Medical nutrition and disease*, 2nd ed. Malden, Massachusetts: Blackwell Science.

Morse, J.M., J.M. Swanson and A.J. Kuzel (eds.) (2001a), *The nature of qualitative evidence.* Thousand Oaks: Sage Publications.

Morse, J.M., J.M. Swanson and A.J. Kuzel (2001b), 'Preface', in: J.M. Morse, J.M. Swanson and A.J. Kuzel (eds.), *The nature of qualitative evidence.* Thousand Oaks: Sage Publications, viii-xiv.

Moss, R.W. (1996), *The cancer industry*, updated ed. Brooklyn, New York: Equinox Press.

Mössinger, P. (1984), *Homöopathie und Naturwissenschaftliche Medizin: zur Ueberwindung der Gegensätze.* Stuttgart: Hippokrates.

Moss-Morris, R., and K.J. Petrie (2000), *Chronic fatigue syndrome.* London: Routledge.

Moyad, M.A. (2001), 'The prevalence and effectiveness of complementary and alternative medicine: what has been learned and what it may be telling us about our patients, ourselves, and conventional medical treatment', *Seminars in urologic oncology*, 19: 257-269.

Moynihan, R. (2003), 'The making of a disease: female sexual dysfunction', *British medical journal*, 326: 4547.

Mueller, P.S., D.J. Plevak and T.A. Rummans (2001), 'Religious involvement, spirituality, and medicine: implications for clinical practice', *Mayo Clinic proceedings* 76: 1225-1235.

Muller, N., M. Riedel, R. Gruber, M. Ackenheil and M.J. Schwarz (2000), 'The immune system and schizophrenia: an integrative view', *Annals of the New York Academy of Science*, 917: 456-467.

Munoz, V., M. Sauvain, G. Bourdy, S. Arrazola, J. Callapa, G. Ruiz, J. Choque and E. Deharo (2000a), 'A search for natural bioactive compounds in Bolivia through a multidisciplinary approach. Part III. Evaluation of the antimalarial activity of plants used by Altenos Indians', *Journal of ethnopharmacology*, 71: 123-131.

Munoz V., M. Sauvain, G. Bourdy, J. Callapa, S. Bergeron, I. Rojas, J.A. Bravo, L. Balderrama, B. Ortiz, A. Gimenez and E. Deharo (2000b), 'A search for natural bioactive compounds in Bolivia through a multidisciplinary approach. Part I. Evaluation of the antimalarial activity of plants used by the Chacobo Indians', *Journal of ethnopharmacology*, 69: 27-37.

Muskin, P.R. (ed.) (2000), *Complementary and alternative medicine and psychiatry.* Washington, D.C.: American Psychiatric Press.

Mustofa, V.A., F. Benoit-Vical, Y. Pelissier, D. Kone-Bamba and M. Mallie (2000), 'Antiplasmodial activity of plant extracts used in west African traditional medicine', *Journal of ethnopharmacology*, 73: 145-151.

Narayanan, B.A., N.K. Narayanan and B.S. Reddy (2001), 'Docosahexaenoic acid regulated genes and transcription factors inducing apoptosis in human colon cancer cells', *International journal of oncology*, 19: 1255-1262.

Nardino, R.J., R.J. Vender and P.N. Herbert (2000), 'Overuse of acid-suppressive therapy in hospitalized patients', *American journal of gastroenterology*, 95: 3118-3122.

Nasir, L. (2000), 'Acupuncture in a university hospital', in: P.B. Fontanarosa (ed.), *Alternative medicine: an objective assessment*. American Medical Association, JAMA and Archives / Journals, 492-496.

Natarajan, S., D. Williamson, J. Grey, K.G. Harding and R.A. Cooper (2001), 'Healing of an MRSA-colonized, hydroxyurea-induced leg ulcer with honey', *Journal of dermatological treatment*, 12: 33-36.

Nelkin, D., and M.S. Lindee (1995), *The DNA mystique: the gene as a cultural icon.* New York: Freeman.

Nelkin, N. (1996), *Consciousness and the origin of thought.* Cambridge:

Cambridge University Press.

Nesse, R.M., and G.C. Williams (1994), *Why we get sick.* New York: Times Books.

Nesse, R.M., and G.C. Williams (1998), 'Evolution and the origins of disease', *Scientific American*, November: 58-65.

Nestle, M. (2002), *Food politics: how the food industry influences nutrition and health.* Berkeley: University of California Press.

Newberg, A., E. D'Aquili and V. Rause (2001), *Why God won't go away.* New York: Random House.

Nikkila, H.V., K. Muller, A. Ahokas, R. Rimon, and L.C. Andersson (2001), 'Increased frequency of activated lymphocytes in the cerebrospinal fluid of patients with acute schizophrenia', *Schizophrenia research*, 49: 99-105.

Nordoy, A., R. Marchioli, H. Arnesen and J. Videbaek (2001), 'N-3 polyunsaturated fatty acids and cardiovascular diseases', *Lipids*, 36, Supplement: S127-S129.

Normark, B.H., and S. Normark (2002), 'Evolution and spread of antibiotic resistance', *Journal of internal medicine*, 252: 91-106.

Nosten, F., and P. Brasseur (2002), 'Combination therapy for malaria: the way forward?', *Drugs*, 62: 1315-1329.

Nzerue, C.M., H. Demissochew and J.K. Tucker (2002), 'Race and kidney disease: role of social and environmental factors', *Journal of the National Medical Association*, 94, Supplement 8: S28-S38.

O'Brien, M. (2000), *Making better environmental decisions: an alternative to risk assessment.* Cambridge, Massachusetts: MIT Press.

O'Connor, B.B. (1995), *Healing traditions: alternative medicine and the health professions.* Philadelphia: University of Pennsylvania Press.

Oketch-Rabah, H.A., J.W. Mwangi, J. Lisgarten and E.K. Mberu (2000), 'A new antiplasmodial coumarin from Toddalia asiatica roots', *Fitoterapia*, 71: 636-640.

Orbach, I. (1995), *The hidden mind: psychology, psychotherapy and unconscious processes.* Chichester: John Wiley & Sons.

Oyama, S., P.E. Griffiths and R.D. Gray (2001), *Cycles of contingency: developmental systems and evolution.* Cambridge, Massachusetts: MIT Press.

Packard, R.M. (1998), 'No other logical choice: global malaria eradication and the politics of international health in the post-war era', *Parasitologia*, 40: 217-229.

Patrick, W.K. (2000), 'Global health challenges: trends in public health training, research and advocacy', *Asia Pacific journal of public health*, 12, Supplement: S8-S12.

Pearsall, P.K. (2001), 'On a wish and a prayer: healing through distant intentionality', *Hawaii medical journal*, 60: 255-256.

Pearce, B.D. (2003), *Can a virus cause schizophrenia? Facts and hypotheses.* Boston: Kluwer.

Peet, M., J. Brind, C.N. Ramchand, S. Shah and G.K. Vankar (2001), 'Two double-blind placebo-controlled pilot studies of eicosapentaenoic acid in the treatment of schizophrenia', *Schizophrenia research*, 49: 243-251.

Peet, M., and D.F. Horrobin (2002)', A dose-ranging exploratory study of the effects of ethyl-eicosapentaenoate in patients with persistent schizophrenic symptoms', *Journal of psychiatric research*, 36: 7-18.

Peet, M., J.D. Laugharne, J. Mellor and C.N. Ramchand (1996), 'Essential fatty acid deficiency in erythrocyte membranes from chronic schizophrenic patients, and the clinical effects of dietary supplementation', *Prostaglandins, leukotrienes, and essential fatty acids*, 55: 71-75.

Pelletier, K. (2000), *The best alternative medicine: what works?, what does not?* New York: Simon & Schuster.

Persinger, M.A. (1987), *Neuropsychological bases of God beliefs.* New York: Praeger.

Peskar, B.M., N. Maricic, B. Gretzera, R. Schuligoi and A. Schmassmann (2001), 'Role of cyclooxygenase-2 in gastric mucosal defense', *Life sciences*, 69: 2993-3003.

Phillimore, P., S. Moffatt, E. Hudson and D. Downey (2000), 'Pollution, politics, and uncertainty: environmental epidemiology in North-East England', in: S. Kroll-Smith, P. Brown and F.J. Guter (eds.), *Illness and the environment: a reader in contested medicine.* New York: New York University Press, 217-234.

Phillips, H. (2003), 'Heart-stopping', *New scientist,* 2377: 36-39.

Pillemer, S.R. (ed.) (1994), *The fibromyalgia syndrome: current research and future directions in epidemiology, pathogenesis, and treatment.* New York: Haworth Medical Press.

Pilotto, A., and P. Malfertheiner (2002), 'Review article: an approach to *Helicobacter pylori* infection in the elderly', *Alimentary pharmacological therapy*, 16: 683-691.

Pincus, T.P. (2002), 'Limitations of randomized clinical trials in chronic diseases: explanations and recommendations', *Advances in mind-body medicine*, 18: 14-21.

Polivy, J., and C.P. Herman (2002), 'Eating disorders', *Annual review of psychology*, 53: 187-213.

Pradalier, A., P. Bakouche, G. Baudesson, A. Delage, G. Cornaille-Lafage, J.M. Launay and P. Biason (2001), 'Failure of omega-3 polyunsaturated fatty acids in prevention of migraine: a double-blind study versus placebo', *Cephalalgia*, 21: 818-822.

Price, D.D., and L.V. Soerensen (2002), 'Endogenous opioid and non-opioid pathways as mediators of placebo analgesia', in: H.A. Guess, A. Kleinman, J.W. Kusek and L.W. Engel (eds.), *The science of the placebo: toward an interdisciplinary research agenda.* London: BMJ Books, 183-206.

Price-Smith, A.T. (2002), *The health of nations: infectious disease, environmental change, and their effects on national security and development.* Cambridge, Massachusetts: MIT Press.

Puri, B.K., G.M. Bydder, S.J. Counsell, B.J. Corridan, A.J. Richardson, J.V. Hajnal, C. Appel, H.M. McKee, K.S. Vaddadi and D.F. Horrobin (2002), 'MRI and neuropsychological improvement in Huntington disease following ethyl-EPA treatment', *Neuroreport*, 13: 123-126.

Puri, B.K., S.J. Counsell, G. Hamilton, A.J. Richardson and D.F. Horrobin (2001), 'Eicosapentaenoic acid in treatment-resistant depression associated with symptom remission, structural brain changes and reduced neuronal phospholipid turnover', *International journal of clinical practice*, 55: 560-563.

Qasim, A., and C.A. O'Morain (2002), 'Review article: treatment of *Helicobacter pylori* infection and factors influencing eradication', *Alimentary pharmacological therapy*, 16, Supplement 1: S24-S30.

Rabin, B.S. (1999), *Stress, immune function, and health: the connection.* New York: John Wiley & Sons.

Raff, R.A. (1996), *The shape of life: genes, development, and the evolution of animal form.* Chicago: University of Chicago Press.

Ravnskov, U. (2000), *The cholesterol myths: exposing the fallacy that saturated fat and cholesterol cause heart disease.* Washington, D.C.: New Trends Publishing Co.

Ray, L.D., and M. Mayan (2001), 'Who decides what counts as evidence?', in: J.M. Morse, J.M. Swanson and A.J. Kuzel (eds.), *The nature of qualitative evidence.* Thousand Oaks: Sage Publications, 50-73.

Reid, G.J., and P.J. McGrath (1996), 'Psychological treatments for migraine', *Biomedicine and pharmacotherapy*, 50: 58-63.

Reynaert, H., E. Fernandes, C. Bourgain, L. Smekens and G. Devis (1995), 'Proton-pump inhibition and gastric giardiasis: a causal or casual association?', *Journal of gastroenterology*, 30: 775-778.

Richardson, A.J., T. Easton, J.H. Gruzelier and B.K. Puri (1999), 'Laterality changes accompanying symptom remission in schizophrenia following treatment with eicosapentaenoic acid', *International journal of psychophysiology*, 34: 333-339.

Richardson, K. (1999), *The making of intelligence.* London: Weidenfeld &

Nicolson.

Richardson, R.C. (1996), 'Critical notice: Robert N. Brandon, adaptation and environment', *Philosophy of science*, 63: 122-136.

Rief, W., F. Pilger, D. Ihle, E. Bosmans, B. Egyed and M. Maes (2001), 'Immunological differences between patients with major depression and somatization syndrome', *Psychiatry research*, 105 : 165-174.

Roberts, A.H. (1994), '"The powerful placebo" revisited: implications for headache treatment and management', *Headache quarterly, current treatment and research*, 5: 208-213.

Roberts, A.H. (1995), 'The powerful placebo revisited: magnitude of nonspecific effects', *Mind-body medicine*, 1: 35-43.

Root-Bernstein, R. and M. Root-Bernstein (1997), *Honey, mud, maggots, and other medical marvels: the science behind folk remedies and old wives' tales.* Boston and New York: Houghton Mifflin Company.

Rose, H., and S. Rose (eds.) (2000), *Alas poor Darwin: arguments against evolutionary psychology*. London: Jonathan Cape.

Ross, C.A., and A. Pam (1995), *Pseudoscience in biological psychiatry: blaming the body*. New York: John Wiley & Sons.

Rothermundt, M., V. Arolt, J. Fenker, H. Gutbrodt, M. Peters and H. Kirchner (2001), 'Different immune patterns in melancholic and non-melancholic major depression', *European archives of psychiatry and clinical neuroscience*, 251: 90-97.

Rothman, D., P. DeLuca and R.B. Zurier (1995), 'Botanical lipids: effects on inflammation, immune responses, and rheumatoid arthritis', *Seminars in arthritis and rheumatism*, 25: 87-96.

Rushton, J.P. (1997), *Race, evolution and behavior.* New Brunswick: Transaction Publishers.

Russell, I.J. (ed.) (1996), *Clinical overview and pathogenesis of the fibromyalgia syndrome, myofascial pain syndrome, and other pain syndromes.* New York: Haworth Medical Press.

Russell, J., L.A. Bau, P.J. Beumont, S. Byrnes, G. Gross, S. Touyz, S. Abraham and S. Zipfel (2001), 'Altered energy metabolism in anorexia nervosa, *Psychoneuroendocrinology*, 26: 51-63.

Russell, R.L. (1994), *Reassessing psychotherapy research.* New York and London: Guilford Press.

Rylko-Bauer, B., and P. Farmer (2002), 'Managed care or managed inequality? A call for critiques of market-based medicine', *Medical anthropology quarterly*, 16: 476-502.

Sabom, M. (1998), *Light and death: one doctor's fascinating account of near-death experiences.* Grand Rapids: Zondervan.

Sackett, D.L., W.M. Rosenberg, J.A. Gray, R.B. Haynes and W.S. Richardson (1996), 'Evidence-based medicine: what it is and what it isn't', *British medical journal*, 312: 71-72.

Sacks, O. (1985), *Migraine, revised and expanded.* Berkeley: University of California Press.

Sampson, W., and L. Vaughn (2000), *Science meets alternative medicine: what the evidence says about unconventional treatments.* Amherst, New York: Prometheus Books.

Sarkar, S. (1998), *Genetics and reductionism.* Cambridge: Cambridge University Press.

Saso, L., G. Valentini, M.L. Casini, E. Mattei, L. Braghiroli, G. Mazzanti, C. Panzironi, E. Grippa and B. Silvestrini (1999), 'Inhibition of protein denaturation by fatty acids, bile salts and other natural substances: a new hypothesis for the mechanism of action of fish oil in rheumatic diseases', *Japanese journal of pharmacology*, 79: 89-99.

Saver, J.L., and J. Rabin (1997), 'The neural substrates of religious experience', *Journal of neuropsychiatry and clinical neurosciences*, 9: 498-510.

Schaffner, K.F. (1993), *Discovery and explanation in biology and medicine.* Chicago: University of Chicago Press.

Schapira, M., M.E. Roquet, J. Henrion, J.M. Ghilain, J.M. Maisin and F.

Heller (1996), 'Severe nontyphoidial salmonellosis probably in relation with omeprazole treatment: Report of 2 cases', *Acta gastroenterologica Belgica*, 59: 168-169.

Schlichting, C.D., and M. Pigliucci (1998), *Phenotypic evolution: a reaction norm perspective.* Sunderland, Massachusetts: Sinauer Associates.

Schwartz, W.B. (1998), *Life without disease: the pursuit of medical utopia.* Berkeley: University of California Press.

Schwarz, M.J., S. Chiang, N. Muller, M. Ackenheil (2001), 'T-helper-1 and T-helper-2 responses in psychiatric disorders', *Brain, behavior, and immunity*, 15: 340-370.

Schwarz, M.J., N. Muller, M. Riedel and M. Ackenheil (2001), 'The Th2-hypothesis of schizophrenia: a strategy to identify a subgroup of schizophrenia caused by immune mechanisms', *Medical hypotheses*, 56: 483-486.

Scott, L.V., and T.G. Dinan (1998), 'Vasopressin and the regulation of hypothalamic-pituitary-adrenal axis function: implications for the pathophysiology of depression', *Life sciences*, 62: 1985-1998.

Scriver, C., A.L. Beaudet, W. S. Sly, D. Valle, B. Vogelstein and B. Childs (eds.) (2001), *The metabolic and molecular bases of inherited diseases*, 8th ed. New York: McGraw Hill.

Seager, W. (1999), *Theories of consciousness: an introduction and assessment.* London: Routledge.

Segal, I. (2001), 'The gastro-oesophageal reflux disease complex in sub-Saharan Africa', *European journal of cancer prevention*, 10: 209-212.

Segerstråle, U. (2000), *Defenders of the truth: the battle for science in the sociobiology debate and beyond.* Oxford: Oxford University Press.

Serhan, C.N., and E. Oliw (2001), 'Unorthodox routes to prostanoid formation: new twists in cyclooxygenase-initiated pathways', *Journal of clinical investigation*, 107: 1481-1489.

Sethi, S., O. Ziouzenkova, H. Ni, D.D. Wagner, J. Plutzky and T.N.

Mayadas (2002), 'Oxidized omega-3 fatty acids in fish oil inhibit leukocyte-endothelial interactions through activation of PPAR alpha', *Blood*, 100: 1340-1346.

Shapiro, A.K., and E. Shapiro (1997a), *The powerful placebo: from ancient priest to modern physician.* Baltimore and London: Johns Hopkins University Press.

Shapiro, A.K., and E. Shapiro (1997b), 'The placebo: is it much ado about nothing?', in: A. Harrington (ed.), *The placebo effect: an interdisciplinary exploration.* Cambridge, Massachusetts: Harvard University Press, 12-36.

Shear, J. (ed.) (1997), *Explaining consciousness: the hard problem.* Cambridge, Massachusetts: MIT Press.

Shears, P. (2001), 'Antibiotic resistance in the tropics: epidemiology and surveillance of antimicrobial resistance in the tropics', *Transactions of the Royal Society of Tropical Medicine and Hygiene*, 95: 127-130.

Sheftell, F.D., and S.J. Tepper (2002), 'New paradigms in the recognition and acute treatment of migraine', *Headache*, 42: 58-69.

Shils, M.E., J.A. Olson, M. Shike and A.C. Ross (1999), *Modern nutrition in health and disease*, 9th ed. Philadelphia: Lippincott Williams & Wilkins.

Shimokawa, H. (2001), 'Beneficial effects of eicosapentaenoic acid on endothelial vasodilator functions in animals and humans', *World review of nutrition and dietetics*, 88: 100-108.

Shiotani, A., Z.Z. Nurgalieva, Y. Yamaoka and D.Y. Graham, '*Helicobacter pylori*', *Medical clinics of North America*, 84: 1125-1136.

Shipman, P. (1994), *The evolution of racism: human differences and the use and abuse of science.* New York: Simon & Schuster.

Sica, D.S., A.C. Schoolwerth and T.W. Gehr (2000), 'Pharmacotherapy in congestive heart failure: COX-2 inhibition: a cautionary note in congestive heart failure', *Congestive heart failure*, 6: 272-276.

Siegel, S. (2002), 'Explanatory mechanisms for placebo effects: Pavlovian conditioning', in: H.A. Guess, A. Kleinman, J.W. Kusek and L.W. Engel (eds.), *The science of the placebo: toward an interdisciplinary research agenda.* London: BMJ Books, 133-157.

Silberstein, S.D. (2001), 'Shared mechanisms and comorbidities in neurologic and psychiatric disorders', *Headache*, 41, Supplement 1: S11-S17.

Simopoulos, A.P. (1991), 'Omega-3 fatty acids in health and disease and in growth and development', *American journal of clinical nutrition*, 54: 438-463.

Simopoulos, A.P. (1995a), 'Genetic variation and nutrition, part 1: population differences due to single gene defects and population differences in multifactorial diseases due to polygenic effects', *Nutrition today*, 30: 157-167.

Simopoulos, A.P. (1995b), 'Genetic variation and nutrition, part 2: genetic variation, nutrition, and chronic diseases', *Nutrition today*, 30: 157-167.

Simopoulos, A.P. (1997), 'Omega-3 fatty acids in the prevention-management of cardiovascular disease', *Canadian journal of physiology and pharmacology*, 75: 234-239.

Simopoulos, A.P. (1999), 'Essential fatty acids in health and chronic disease', *American journal of clinical nutrition*, 70, Supplement: S560-S569.

Simopoulos, A.P. (2001a), 'The Mediterranean diets: What is so special about the diet of Greece?', *Journal of nutrition*, 131: S3065-S3073.

Simopoulos, A.P. (2001b), 'N-3 fatty acids and human health: defining strategies for public policy', *Lipids*, 36: 583-589.

Simopoulos, A.P. (2002a), 'Omega-3 fatty acids in inflammation and autoimmune diseases', *Journal of the American College of Nutrition*, 21: 495-505.

Simopoulos, A.P. (2002b), 'The importance of the ratio of omega-6/omega-3 essential fatty acids', *Biomedicine and pharmacotherapy*, 56: 365-379.

Simopoulos, A.P., H.A. Norman and J. Gillaspy (1995), 'Purslane in human nutrition and its potential for world agriculture', *World review of nutrition and dietetics*, 77: 47-74.

Simopoulos, A.P., H.A. Norman, J. Gillaspy and J.A. Duke (1992), 'Common purslane: a source of omega-3 fatty acids and antioxidants', *Journal of the American College of Nutrition*, 11: 374-382.

Simopoulos, A.P., and Salem Jr, N. (1986), 'Purslane: a terrestrial source of omega-3 fatty acids', *New England journal of medicine*, 315: 833.

Singer, B.H., and M.C. de Castro (2001), 'Agricultural colonization and malaria on the Amazon frontier', *Annals of the New York Academy of Science*, 954: 184-222.

Singh, R., S. Gopalan and A. Sibal (2002), 'Immunonutrition', *Indian journal of pediatrics*, 69: 417-419.

Sivakumar, K., and M.C. Dalakas (1994), 'Autoimmune syndrome induced by omeprazole', *Lancet*, 344: 619-620.

Sivik, T., D. Byrne, D. Lipsitt, G. Christodoulou and H. Dienstfrey (2002) (eds.), *Psycho-neuro-endocrino-immunology (PNEI).* Amsterdam: Elsevier.

Skelly, M., and A. Helm (eds.) (1999), *Alternative treatments for fibromyalgia & chronic fatigue syndrome: insights from practitioners and patients.* Alameda: Hunter House Publishers.

Skrabanek, P., and J. McCormick (1989), *Follies and fallacies in medicine.* Glasgow: Tarragon Press.

Slavin, M.O., and D. Kriegman (1992), *The adaptive design of the human psyche: psychoanalysis, evolutionary biology, and the therapeutic process.* New York: Guilford Press.

Sloan, R.P., and E. Bagiella (2002), 'Claims about religious involvement and health outcomes', *Annals of behavioral medicine*, 24: 14-21.

Sloan, R.P., E. Bagiella, L. VandeCreek, M. Hover, C. Casalone, T. Jinpu Hirsch, Y. Hasan, R. Kreger and P. Poulos (2000), 'Should physicians prescribe religious activities?' *The New England journal of medicine*, 342: 1913-1916.

Sloan, R.P., E. Bagiella and T. Powell (1999), 'Religion, spirituality, and medicine', *Lancet*, 353, 664-667.

Smith, R.S. (1992), 'The cytokine theory of headache', *Medical hypotheses*, 39: 168-174.

Soldz, S., and L. McCullough (2000), *Reconciling empirical knowledge and clinical experience.* Washington, D.C.: American Psychological Association.

Sood, A., M. Sharma, N.P. Jain, L.S. Chawla and R. Kumar (1995), 'Esophageal candidiasis following omeprazole therapy: a report of two cases', *Indian journal of gastroenterology*, 14: 71-72.

Sperner-Unterweger, B., W.W. Fleischhacker and W.P. Kaschka (eds.) (2001), *Psychoneuroimmunology: hypotheses and current research.* Basel: Karger.

Spiro, H. (1998), *The power of hope.* New Haven and London: Yale University Press.

Staats, P.S. (2002), 'Pain management and beyond: evolving concepts and treatments involving cyclooxygenase inhibition', *Journal of pain and symptom management*, 24, Supplement 1: S4-S9.

Stalker, C., and C. Glymour (1989), *Examining holistic medicine.* Buffalo, New York: Prometheus Books.

Stanford, C.B. (1999), *The hunting apes: meat eating and the origins of human behavior.* Princeton: Princeton University Press.

Stassi, G., A. Arena, A. Speranza, D. Iannello and P. Mastroeni (2002), 'Different modulation by live or killed *Helicobacter pylori* on cytokine production from peripheral blood mononuclear cells', *The new microbiologica*, 25: 247-252.

Stelfox, H.T., G. Chua, K. O'Rourke and A.S. Detsky (1998), 'Conflict of interest in the debate over calcium-channel antagonists', *The New England journal of medicine*, 338: 101-110.

Stephens, G., and G. Graham (2000), *When self-consciousness breaks: alien voices and inserted thoughts.* Cambridge, Massachusetts: MIT Press.

Sterelny, K., and P.E. Griffiths (1999), *Sex and death: an introduction to the philosophy of biology.* Chicago: University of Chicago Press.

Stevens, A., and J. Price (1996), *Evolutionary psychiatry: a new beginning.* London: Routledge.

Stoll, A.L. (2001), *The omega-3 connection.* New York: Simon & Schuster.

Stompe, T., G. Ortwein-Swoboda, K. Ritter, H. Schanda and A. Friedmann (2002), 'Are we witnessing the disappearance of catatonic schizophrenia?', *Comparative psychiatry*, 43: 167-174.

Su, K.P., S.J. Leu, Y.Y. Yang, W.W. Shen, Y.M. Chou and S.Y. Tsai (2002), 'Reduced production of interferon-gamma but not interleukin-10 in bipolar mania and subsequent remission', *Journal of affective disorders*, 71: 205-209.

Su, K.P., W.W. Shen and S.Y. Huang (2001), 'Omega-3 fatty acids as a psychotherapeutic agent for a pregnant schizophrenic patient', *European neuropsychopharmacology*, 11: 295-299.

Susser, E.S., A.S. Brown and J.M. Gorman (eds.) (1999), *Prenatal exposures in schizophrenia.* Washington, D.C.: American Psychiatric Press.

Swanson, D.R. (1986), 'Fish oil, Raynaud's syndrome, and undiscovered public knowledge', *Perspectives in biology and medicine*, 30: 7-17.

Swanson, D.R. (1987), 'Two medical literatures that are logically but not bibliographically connected', *Journal of the American Society for Information Science*, 38: 228-233.

Swanson, D.R. (1988), 'Migraine and magnesium: eleven neglected connections', *Perspectives in biology and medicine*, 31: 527-557.

Swanson, D.R. (1990), 'Medical literature as a potential source of new knowledge', *Bulletin of the Medical Libraries Association*, 78: 29-37.

Swanson, D.R. (1991), 'Complementary structures in disjoint science literatures', *SIGIR91: proceedings of the 14th annual international ACM.*

Chicago: ACM Press.

Swanson, D.R. (2001), 'ASIST award of merit acceptance speech on the fragmentation of knowledge, the connection explosion, and assembling other people's ideas', *Bulletin of the American Society for Information Science and Technology*, February / March: 12-14.

Swanson, D.R., and N.R. Smalheiser (1997), 'An interactive system for finding complementary literatures: a stimulus to scientific discovery', *Artificial intelligence*, 91: 183-203.

Swanson, D.R., and N.R. Smalheiser (1999), 'Implicit text linkages between Medline records: using Arrowsmith as an aid to scientific discovery', *Library trends*, 48: 48-59.

Swayne, J. (1998), 'Homeopathic therapeutics: many dimensions—or meaningless diversity?' in: A. Vickers (ed.), *Examining complementary medicine.* Cheltenham: Stanley Thornes, 64-73.

Sykes, B. (1999), *The human inheritance: genes, language, and evolution.* Oxford: Oxford University Press.

Tamblyn, R., L. Berkson, W.D. Dauphinee, D. Gayton, R. Grad, A. Huang, L. Isaac, P. McLeod and L. Snell (1997), 'Unnecessary prescribing of NSAIDs and the management of NSAID-related gastropathy in medical practice', *Annals of internal medicine*, 127: 429-438.

Teare, J.P., C. Spedding, M.W. Whitehead, S.M. Greenfield, S.J. Challacombe and R.P. Thompson (1995), 'Omeprazole and dry mouth', *Scandinavian journal of gastroenterology*, 30: 216-218.

Temple, N.J. (2002), 'Nutrition and disease: challenges of research design', *Nutrition*, 18: 343-347.

Terada, S., M. Takizawa, S. Yamamoto, O. Ezaki, H. Itakura and K.S. Akagawa (2001), 'Suppressive mechanisms of EPA on human T cell proliferation', *Microbiology and immunology*, 45: 473-481.

Thagard, P. (1999), *How scientists explain disease*. Princeton: Princeton University Press.

Theisen, J., D. Nehra, D. Citron, J. Johansson, J.A. Hagen, P.F. Crookes,

S.R. DeMeester, C.G. Bremner, T.R. DeMeester and J.H. Peters (2000), 'Suppression of gastric acid secretion in patients with gastroesophageal reflux disease results in gastric bacterial overgrowth and deconjugation of bile acids', *Journal of gastrointestinal surgery*, 4: 50-54.

Thomas, J., W.L. Straus and B.S. Bloom (2002), 'Over-the-counter nonsteroidal anti-inflammatory drugs and risk of gastrointestinal symptoms', *American journal of gastroenterology*, 97: 2215-2219.

Thompson, L., A. Cockayne and R.C. Spiller (1994), 'Inhibitory effect of polyunsaturated fatty acids on the growth of *Helicobacter pylori*: a possible explanation of the effect of diet on peptic ulceration', *Gut*, 35: 1557-1561.

Tona, L., N.P. Ngimbi, M. Tsakala, K. Mesia, K. Cimanga, S. Apers, T. De Bruyne, L. Pieters, J. Totte and A.J. Vlietinck (1999), 'Antimalarial activity of 20 crude extracts from nine African medicinal plants used in Kinshasa, Congo', *Journal of ethnopharmacology*, 68: 193-203.

Tovey, F.I., and M. Hobsley (1998), 'Clarification of the link between polyunsaturated fatty acids and *Helicobacter pylori*-associated duodenal ulcer disease: a dietary intervention study', *British journal of nutrition*, 80: 116-117.

Tovey, F.I., and M. Hobsley (1999), 'Is *Helicobacter pylori* the primary cause of duodenal ulceration?', *Journal of gastroenterology and hepatology*, 14: 1053-1056.

Trape, J.F., G. Pison, A. Spiegel, C. Enel and C. Rogier (2002), 'Combating malaria in Africa', *Trends in parasitology*, 18: 224-230.

Trust, T.J., R.A. Alm and J. Pappo (2001), '*Helicobacter pylori*: today's treatment, and possible future treatment', *European journal of surgery*, Supplement (586): S82-S88.

Ulak, G., R. Cicek, A. Sermet, C. Guzel, M. Ulak and O. Denli (1995), 'Protective effect of fish oil against stress-induced gastric injury in rats', *Arzneimittelforschung*, 45: 1174-1175.

Upshur, R.E.G. (2001), 'The status of qualitative research as evidence', in: J.M. Morse, J.M. Swanson and A.J. Kuzel (eds.), *The nature of qualitative evidence.* Thousand Oaks: Sage Publications, 5-26.

Uttal, W.R. (2001), *The new phrenology: the limits of localizing cognitive processes in the brain.* Cambridge, Massachusetts: MIT Press.

Van der Steen, W.J. (1993a), *A practical philosophy for the life sciences.* Albany: State University of New York Press.

Van der Steen, W.J. (1993b), 'Towards a practicable methodology for medicine: the impact of conceptual analysis', *Perspectives in biology and medicine*, 36: 580-591.

Van der Steen, W.J. (1995), *Facts, values, and methodology: a new approach to ethics*. Amsterdam: Rodopi.

Van der Steen, W.J. (1999a), 'Bias in behavior genetics: an ecological perspective', *Acta biotheoretica*, 46: 369-377.

Van der Steen, W.J. (1999b), 'Parallels between science and ethics', in: A.W. Musschenga and W.J. van der Steen (eds.), *Reasoning in ethics and the law: theory, principle, and judgment.* Aldershot: Ashgate.

Van der Steen, W.J. (2000a), *Evolution as natural history: a philosophical analysis.* Westport: Praeger.

Van der Steen, W.J. (2000b), 'Chronic fatigue syndrome: A matter of enzyme deficiencies?', *Medical hypotheses*, 54: 853-854.

Van der Steen, W.J. (2000c), 'Science, religion and experience', *American philosophical quarterly*, 40: 339-349.

Van der Steen, W.J., and V.K.Y. Ho (2001a), *Methods and morals in the life sciences: a guide for analyzing and writing texts.* Westport: Praeger.

Van der Steen, W.J., and V.K.Y. Ho (2001b), 'Drugs versus diets: disillusions with Dutch health care', *Acta biotheoretica*, 49: 125-140.

Van der Steen, W.J., and P.J. Thung (1988), *Faces of medicine: a philosophical study.* Dordrecht: Kluwer.

Van der Weele, C. (1999), *Images of development: environmental causes in ontogeny.* Albany: State University of New York Press.

Vickers, A. (ed.) (1998), *Examining complementary medicine.* Cheltenham: Stanley Thornes.

Villanueva, P., S. Peiro, J. Librero and I. Pereiro (2003), 'Accuracy of pharmaceutical advertisements in medical journals', *Lancet*, 361: 27-32.

Vincent, C., and A. Furnham (1997), *Complementary medicine: a research perspective.* Chichester: John Wiley & Sons.

Volker, D., P. Fitzgerald, G. Major and M. Garg (2000), 'Efficacy of fish oil concentrate in the treatment of rheaumatoid arthritis', *Journal of rheumatology*, 27: 2343-2346.

Voulgari, P.V., Y. Alamanos, D. Papazisi, K. Christou, C. Papanikolaou and A.A. Drosos (2000), 'Prevalence of Raynaud's phenomenon in a healthy Greek population', *Annals of rheumatic diseases*, 59: 206-210.

Wahlbeck, K., and C. Adams (1999), 'Beyond conflict of interest: sponsored drug trials show more favourable outcomes', *British medical journal*, 318: 465.

Waldum, H.L., J.S. Arnestad, E. Brenna, I. Eide and U. Syversen (1996), 'Marked increase in gastric acid secretory capacity after omeprazole treatment', *Gut*, 39: 649-653.

Weiser, M., W, Strösser and P. Klein (2000), 'Homeopathic vs conventional treatment of vertigo: a randomized double-blind controlled clinical study', in: P.B. Fontanarosa (ed.), *Alternative medicine: an objective assessment*. American Medical Association, JAMA and Archives / Journals, 432-440.

Willcox, M.L. (1999), 'A clinical trial of 'AM', a Ugandan herbal remedy for malaria', *Journal of public health and medicine*, 21: 318-324.

Williams, B. (2002), *Surviving "terminal" cancer: clinical trials, drug cocktails & other treatments your oncologist won't tell you about.* Minneapolis: Fairview Press.

Wolfe, M.M. (1996), 'NSAIDs and the gastrointestinal mucosa', *Hospital practice*, 31: 37-44, 47-48.

Wongsrichanalai, C., A.L. Pickard, W.H. Wernsdorfer and S.R. Meshnick

(2002), 'Epidemiology of drug-resistant malaria', *Lancet infectious diseases*, 2: 209-218.

Woodward, M., H. Tunstall-Pedoe and K. McColl (2001), '*Helicobacter pylori* infection reduces systemic availability of dietary vitamin C', *European journal of gastroenterology and hepatology*, 13: 233-237.

Yamada, N., J. Shimizu J, M. Wada, T. Takita, and S. Innami (1998), 'Changes in platelet aggregation and lipid metabolism in rats given dietary lipids containing different n-3 polyunsaturated fatty acids', *Journal of nutritional science and vitaminology*, (Tokyo) 44: 279-289.

Yao, J.K., R.D. Reddy and D.P. van Kammen (2001), 'Oxidative damage and schizophrenia: an overview of the evidence and its therapeutic implications', *CNS drugs*, 15: 287-310.

Zhang, X.Y., D.F. Zhou, P.Y. Zhang, G.Y. Wu, L.Y. Cao and Y.C Shen (2002), 'Elevated interleukin-2, interleukin-6 and interleukin-8 serum levels in neuroleptic-free schizophrenia: association with psychopathology', *Schizophrenia research*, 57: 247-258.

Zhu, A.J., and B.T. Walsh (2002), 'Pharmacologic treatment of eating disorders', *Canadian journal of psychiatry*, 47: 227-234.

Zillmer, E.A., and M. Spiers (2001), *Principles of neuropsychology.* Belmont: Wadsworth/Thomson Learning.

Zingrone, N.L. (2002), 'Controversy and the problems of parapsychology', *The journal of parapsychology*, 66: 3-30.

Zuckerman, M. (1999), *Vulnerability to psychopathology: a biosocial model.* Washington, D.C.: American Psychological Association.

Author Index

Subject Index